Disorders of Human Learning, Behavior, and Communication

Ronald L. Taylor and Les Sternberg
Series Editors

D1713860

Glenn Affleck   Howard Tennen
Jonelle Rowe

Infants in Crisis

How Parents Cope
with Newborn Intensive Care
and Its Aftermath

With 17 Illustrations

Springer-Verlag
New York Berlin Heidelberg London
Paris Tokyo Hong Kong Barcelona

Glenn Affleck, Professor of Psychiatry, School of Medicine, The University of Connecticut Health Center, Farmington, CT 06032, USA

Howard Tennen, Department of Psychiatry, School of Medicine, The University of Connecticut Health Center, Farmington, CT 06032, USA

Jonelle Rowe, Department of Pediatrics, School of Medicine, The University of Connecticut Health Center, Farmington, CT 06032, USA

Series Editors: Ronald L. Taylor and Les Sternberg, Exceptional Student Education, Florida Atlantic University, Boca Raton, FA 33431-0991, USA

Library of Congress Cataloging-in-Publication Data
Affleck, Glenn.
  Infants in Crisis : how parents cope with newborn intensive care and its aftermath / Glenn
    Affleck, Howard Tennen, Jonelle Rowe. p.   cm—(Disorders of human learning,
    behavior, and communication)
  Includes bibliographical references.
  Includes indexes.
  ISBN 0-387-97392-3 (alk. paper).—ISBN 3-540-97392-3 (alk. paper)
 ·1. Neonatal intensive care—Psychological aspects.   2. Parent and
child.   3. Adjustment (Psychology)   4. Infants (Newborn)—Family
relationships.   I. Tennen, Howard.   II. Rowe, Jonelle C.
III. Title.   IV. Series.
  [DNLM: 1. Adaptation, Psychological.   2. Infant, Newborn, Diseases.
3. Intensive Care, Neonatal.   4. Life-Change Events   5. Parent–Child
Relations.   WS 420 A257c]
RJ253.5.A35   1991
155.9′16—dc20
DNLM/DLC
for Library of Congress   90-10101

Printed on acid-free paper.

Typeset by Best-Set Typesetters, Ltd., Chai Wan, Hong Kong.
Printed and bound by R.R. Donnelley and Sons, Harrisonburg, VA.
Printed in the United States of America.

9 8 7 6 5 4 3 2 1

ISBN 0-387-97392-3 Springer-Verlag New York Berlin Heidelberg
ISBN 3-540-97392-3 Springer-Verlag Berlin Heidelberg New York

Dedicated to our families, and theirs

Preface

More than 10 years ago, with funding from the Connecticut State Department of Education and the encouragement of its consultant on early childhood special education, Virginia Volk, we began our studies of families of infants who were hospitalized on the newborn intensive care unit of the John Dempsey Hospital located at the University of Connecticut Health Center. Betty Jo McGrade, Deborah Allen, and Maria McQueeney played pivotal roles in the early years of this research program. Additional funding from the National March of Dimes Foundation, the University of Connecticut Research Foundation, and the National Institute of Mental Health prepared the ground for the study we describe in this book.

The study began in 1984 through a National Institute of Disability and Rehabilitation Research center grant to the University of Connecticut Pediatric Research and Training Center, directed by Robert Greenstein and then by Mary Beth Bruder. Linda Walker coordinated the project and conducted the interviews with families before hospital discharge. Pamela Higgins conducted all follow-up interviews and assisted with data management and analysis. Elizabeth Trueb Roscher provided support services to a portion of the families who were studied. Deborah Begin transcribed interviews and handled the administrative details of the project. Richard Mendola was the consultant on data analysis and the selection of computer software and hardware.

To all these individuals we extend our deepest gratitude for their contributions to this book. We are also deeply indebted to the medical and nursing staff of John Dempsey Hospital's Newborn Intensive Care Unit for their continued support of our research on the psychosocial aspects of newborn intensive care. But we reserve our warmest thanks to the mothers and fathers who so generously gave their time and energies to make this book a reality. In what was a difficult and demanding time, they opened their homes and their hearts in the hope that they could teach professionals and inspire parents who found themselves in similar circumstances. We hope that we have done them justice in our efforts to chronicle their experiences.

Glenn Affleck
Howard Tennen
Jonelle Rowe

Contents

1
Introduction

Before describing the plan of this book and the background and details of our study, we will allow our informants to speak to the reader in their own words. We begin this way because it was our in-depth interviews with parents that taught us the most about the psychological threats and challenges of the unfolding crisis of newborn intensive care. It was through these interviews that we began to understand the phenomenology of this stressful event. A natural beginning to our analysis of parents' adaptation to the birth, hospitalization, and homecoming of medically fragile infants is to understand how these events threaten patents' well-being and challenge their social and psychological resources.

The Psychological Challenges of Newborn Intensive Care

The Birth and Delivery

The mother quoted below offered a characteristic account of the escalating crisis of her baby's delivery, 3 months early:

> My pregnancy was great. I had no morning sickness. I felt fine and had a lot of energy. I never missed a day's work. I had been doing everything to make sure that things would turn out all right. Then one night while we were getting ready to go out to dinner, I went into the bathroom, and all of a sudden, blood was pouring out of me. My husband called the doctor, who said I should go to the hospital right away, which we did. Then the doctor had me transferred to the medical center where they hooked me up to IVs and monitors. They weren't willing to wait, so they delivered the baby by C section. And only 4 hours earlier, I had been thinking about going out to dinner. That's what was so weird about it... that it happened so suddenly, without any warning.

Like 70% of the mothers who participated in our study, this woman had no warning of a premature or hazardous delivery. Her pregnancy had been proceeding uneventfully, and she had been doing all the "right" things to make sure it would stay that way. Yet, her expectations were abruptly violated.

This response to the birth of a premature or sick newborn—a sense of dashed expectations and shattered assumptions—echoes the reaction of people who encounter other upsetting and unexpected events: becoming seriously ill, losing a loved one, being the victim of criminal assault, or surviving a natural disaster. Contributors to the rapidly growing literature on the psychology of victimization agree that one of the most powerful threats to victims' well-being is that they challenge cherished beliefs, even "illusions," about ourselves and the world (Janoff-Bulman & Frieze, 1983; Taylor, 1983; Taylor & Brown, 1988). Janoff-Bulman (1989) writes, "the psychological disequilibrium and emotional upheaval experienced by victims is largely a reflection of this intense, serious challenge to their basic assumptions. . . All of sudden victims are confronted with a world that is malevolent and meaningless, and a view of themselves as having been singled out for misfortune" (p. 163).

Janoff-Bulman and Frieze (1983) remind us that we "from day to day. . .operate on the basis of assumptions and personal theories that allow [us] to set goals, plan activities, and order [our] behavior" (p. 3). Our "assumptive world" (Parkes, 1975), or what Thompson and Janigian (1988) call our "life scheme" and what Bowlby (1969) calls our "world models," includes the tendency to see ourselves as having control over events, to view ourselves as relatively invulnerable, to regard the things that happen to us as being orderly, predictable, and meaningful, and to see ourselves as worthy and others as benevolent or at least benign.

The centrality of these assumptions in our lives is revealed most starkly when we face a personal catastrophe that challenges their validity. Consider, for example, the common perception that "bad things happen, but not to me." This illusion, which Perloff (1983) calls a sense of *unique* invulnerability, is comforting because it allows us to live from day to day without feeling overwhelmed by the possibility of danger and harm. Often, a belief in personal invulnerability is buttressed by the conviction that we can prevent bad things from happening. These twin assumptions are usually so robust that they go unquestioned in the face of minor disappointments and misfortunes. Only traumatic events bring them to light.

Does the birth of a medically fragile newborn threaten the validity of parents' valued assumptions? One set of findings that begin to answer this question concerns mothers' expectations about the outcome of their pregnancy and their efforts to prevent complications of pregnancy and delivery. Approximately half the mothers who participated in our study said that when they were pregnant they had imagined that there was no possibility that their baby would need to be hospitalized on a newborn intensive care unit (NICU). Only a small handful of the mothers, most of whom had been through this before with other children, had thought that there was a better than even chance that this would happen to them.

Virtually all of these mothers recounted things that they had done during their pregnancy to prevent such problems from occurring. The vast majority said that they had made changes in their habits and lifestyle—avoiding alcohol, quitting smoking, following a more nutritious diet, exercising more, and trying to reduce the stress in their lives. One in four mothers quit their jobs and the same number quit taking all medications. Most of the fathers we interviewed also identified ways in which they had helped their wives to ensure an uneventful pregnancy. Nearly half these men said that they took on greater responsibilities for housework and childcare to make things easier for their wives, and about 20% said they tried to provide more emotional support than usual to enhance their wives' psychological well-being.

Many mothers and fathers volunteered how this event had violated their expectations of control over the pregnancy:

> I really thought everything was going to be fine. I couldn't imagine anything would go wrong. I was very good with my pregnancy. I exercised. I didn't smoke or drink. I followed all of the advice in the books.

> My wife was particular about what she ate and took extra good care of herself. So I can't understand why it happened. There was simply no reason for it.

> I can't understand it. I did everything I was supposed to. I didn't drink, I didn't smoke, I quit work, I followed my doctor's advice. This was not supposed to happen.

> This is something I thought would never happen to me. I waited all my life to have a baby. I expected it to be a joyful experience. I did everything to prepare for a happy time. There was no reason to think anything would go wrong. It just doesn't make any sense.

> I kept asking why? We don't deserve this. We did everything right. . . watched every meal, did every exercise. . . just to make sure that everything would be perfect. And, then, in a matter of hours, something like this happens to turn your whole world upside down.

Some parents, instead of questioning their expectations of personal control, questioned the control they had accorded to their obstetrician. One parent's conclusion that the obstetrician was to blame for the child's medical problems was framed by assumptions about this physician's ability, but failure, to control the outcome of the pregnancy:

> What happened to my child simply should not have happened. If he was born deformed, that's one thing. But my son's problem is something that could have been prevented and should have been prevented. He missed something. He knew better. I don't think I'll ever get over this fact.

Finally, in addition to shattering expectations of invulnerability and control, the crisis of newborn intensive care caused some parents to question the meaningfulness, even fairness, of events:

> Of all the people in the world, why did this happen to me? Why not someone else? Things don't make sense any more.

How could God do this to us? I'm mad as hell. Why now? Why us? Why was my baby going through all of this ? What did he do to deserve this? I've lived my life. Let me suffer instead.

It's just not fair. Here I did everything I was supposed to do. And this woman in the bed next to me, who was a heavy smoker, had this moose of a kid. So why me and not her?

The Hospitalization

Many authors have identified the stresses faced by parents whose new-borns are hospitalized on a NICU (e.g., Bogdan, Brown, & Foster, 1982; Briggs, 1985; Pederson, Bento, Chance, Evans, & Fox, 1987; Silcock, 1984). They have commented on the baby's life and death struggle, the chaotic intensive care environment, painful treatment procedures, conflicts with treatment staff, difficult treatment choices, and the child's uncertain prognosis. Many of these challenges were represented in parents' own descriptions of their child's hospitalization on the unit.

This phase of the crisis begins when a parent sees the infant in the NICU for the first time. Many mothers recounted this distressing encounter in dramatic terms:

I wasn't really sad or scared the first time I saw him. . .just kind of numb and confused. His head was so small, I felt I could crush it by just touching it.

The picture I had of him in my mind did not portray what he actually looked like. He looked like those starving babies you see in Africa. . .all skin and bones.

I just couldn't believe my eyes. He didn't look like he was real. His rear end didn't have any cheeks, just a tiny line. His thighs were like my baby finger. I couldn't believe that anything that small could live.

The first time I saw him, he was beet red and transparent. He looked strangely like a newborn kitten. His eyes were fused shut. He didn't look real.

When I first saw him, it was weird. I thought to myself, "this isn't my child. He isn't going to look like me or my husband." Actually he didn't even look like a person. He was this tiny creature with tubes.

I walked into the unit, and there she was. . .hooked up to all these machines. I just stood there. It could have been for hours. People were saying things to me, but I didn't hear a word.

It was like a dream. . .no, a nightmare. I was saying, "this is not me, this is not my baby."

They took me up to the nursery in a wheelchair. There she was, bright red, lying on a big table. The way she was lying, it reminded me of Jesus on the cross.

The imagery used by these mothers reveals both the emotional distancing and the unreality that accompanied them on their first visit to the NICU. Unable, perhaps unwilling, to fell an immediate affection for their child, many then chronicled the difficulties they faced in becoming emotionally attached to their baby in the hospital.

> Right from the beginning, I didn't feel like I was bonded to her. I never felt that she was mine. I worried that she and I would never really love each other.

> I remember deciding not to visit for a while. The reason I said was that I had a cold. But really, I was happy to have a reason not to go. . . not so much because I didn't care about her, but because I just didn't want to be attached to a child who was less than I wanted her to be.

> Looking back on it, I just didn't want to accept him as my child. The doctors were telling us that his chances weren't too good. I didn't want to become attached and then have my heart broken.

Almost half the mothers mentioned their child's uncertain survival as the most difficult part of this experience. Many, such as those quoted next, described an almost constant fear that their baby could die at any moment:

> There was this deep and awful fear that no matter how much they did for him, he could die the very next minute. So, every time we went into the unit, we were scared to death.

> The first 2 weeks were the hardest. I honestly didn't know if he was going to live or die. Every time the phone would ring, I would jump out of my skin, fearing the bad news had finally come.

> The doctors never knew what would happen next. One day things were good, the next day they were bad. You didn't know whether to feel relieved or to prepare yourself for his death.

One in 10 mothers identified the environment of the NICU as the most difficult aspect of their child's hospitalization. Relatively few parents said that they had had any direct exposure to intensive care for adults, let alone infants. As one mother said, "I knew babies were born early, but I never stopped to think about what happened to them after the delivery." Not surprisingly, then, several described the unit as an alien world, where nothing normal or familiar seemed to happen.

> When you walk onto the unit, it's like walking into an iron lung. You have trouble breathing. It's also like being in an *Alice in Wonderland* nightmare. It's a strange world, with its own atmosphere, different even from the rest of the hospital. The reality is that babies are dying here, but you can't cope with that. So, an artificial world is set up where people live by artificial rules.

> That whole place is very scary and crazy. There's people running all over the place. And all those machines! There's nothing normal about it, nothing at all.

> The unit was overwhelming because of all the equipment needed to keep the babies alive. It made us see our baby as so fragile that we hesitated to touch her for the longest time. It is really a very different world in there.

> The thing that frightened me most was to see all the babies hooked up to machines. You look around and say to yourself, "this does not look good." I

would take her into the family room as often as I could because I just couldn't stand seeing and hearing those machines.

Looking back on this experience, many mothers also expressed regret that they were unable to assume their full role as caregivers. One third of the mothers viewed this as the most disturbing aspect of newborn intensive care:

I didn't really feel like a mother at all. I couldn't have him with me and do what other mothers do. Something was missing. Everyone was congratulating me, but I couldn't understand what they meant. What was there to congratulate?

What was hardest was to surrender the care of your child to someone else, in fact, to many people. I had prepared for months to take care of this child, but then it was taken away from me, by the situation.

Ten percent of the mothers described the most difficult characteristic of this situation as a more general feeling of helplessness:

All the time he was in the hospital, I was in a state of limbo...suspended in time and space. There was just no control I could have over what was happening. I didn't even pray because I didn't think that would help either.

I felt completely helpless. There was nothing I could do to make a difference. It was nothing I knew anything about. So I felt at the total mercy of events I couldn't influence.

I felt as if the whole experience took 20 years off my life. It was a feeling of complete helplessness. Here I am having produced this baby and I don't even have the power to keep it alive. It's been a very powerful awakening to feel that I can't control destiny. I like to feel in control of things, and to feel helpless is a very painful experience.

Finally, 10% of the mothers called their child's uncertain prognosis the most threatening aspect of this experience. Several parents found themselves worrying about the possibility that their child might end up severely disabled:

I found myself thinking about the possibility that my child might be handicapped. I would think about how handicapped children are different. I know that you can give them the love and care they need. But those storybook images of my child may never come true.

They told us that if she didn't die that she might have severe disabilities or be retarded. I began to envision terrible things that you see in the newspapers or on TV...children who have to be spoonfed and the like.

The Transition Home

We turn next to the challenges mothers encountered in the first few months of caring for their child at home. We should emphasize that the challenges after discharge seemed fewer, generally less intense, and more easily met than those that mothers had described at hospital discharge. Most mothers looked back on the first months after their child's homecoming as a generally satisfying time, especially when they compared this to what they had faced during their child's hospital stay or what they had feared might happen once they took their child home.

When describing the most difficult problem they encountered during the first 6 months after their child's discharge, one in four mothers called attention to their child's continuing medical problems. More specifically, they were distressed by their child's continued dependence on medical technology (e.g., oxygen tanks and apnea monitors) and medications (especially those with behavioral side effects), poor weight gain, and recurrent illnesses.

> The worst thing was when he came down with bronchitis and had to go back into the hospital for 10 days. I thought to myself that he really will die now.

> For the first 3 months, he had to be on oxygen for 3 hours a day. That would make him very fussy. And it was almost impossible to keep that mask taped to his face. We had to bring him to the hospital when he got the flu. They put him in an oxygen tent and it was like everything was starting all over again.

A second difficulty, cited as often as continuing medical problems, was the exhausting routine of caring for the infant. In this category, mothers referred to their own lack of sleep from the baby's unpredictable sleep schedule, their frustration over feeding problems, their inability to find techniques to calm their baby's crying and distress, and other caregiving problems.

> He is constant work from the minute he gets up in the morning. And there's just no consistency. For a time, he starts to sleep well and then he goes into a period when he doesn't seem to sleep at all. I can't tell what he wants to eat or even if he wants to eat at all.

> He's often irritable and won't sleep well. There was a time when he would cry for hours in the middle of the night.

> I've been afraid to take him anywhere, because the minute he gets there he starts crying inconsolably.

> Sometimes it felt like she would cry for weeks without stopping. Any time we took her somewhere, she would start, and there was nothing I could do to stop it.

A third difficulty, reported by about 10% of the mothers, stemmed from their perception of the child as fragile and needing special protection. Several expressed a fear of leaving their child in the care of others. Yet, they were reluctant to take their child out of the house, for fear of exposing him or her to infection. These and other mothers commented on the first weeks home as a time of extreme anxiety over whether the baby might still die without warning:

For awhile, we were so scared that we both slept on the couch near her cradle. I thought she would stop breathing. I had heard that babies like this have a greater chance of crib death. Some nights I wouldn't sleep at all just watching her sleep and listening for her breathing.

The mother quoted next made extraordinary accommodations in the home environment and family routines arising out of concern for her infant's physical well-being:

When she first came home, I was terribly afraid. The biggest thing they tell you is that these children have weak lungs and are susceptible to lung infections. So before she came home I had all the rugs and carpets washed. I wouldn't let anyone come into the house. I wouldn't even let anyone come close enough to breathe on her. I guess I became accustomed to the sterile atmosphere of the NICU. I became obsessed with protecting her. Because I couldn't go out of the house, I was feeling like a prisoner in my own home.

A final difficulty, described by 15% of the mothers, concerned conflicts in relationships with family, friends, and professionals over the perception and care of the child. Differing opinions of the child's need for special protection was the subject of debate in many of the extended families. Another key source of tension in the family was the inability to reconcile differing views of the child's progress. Some mothers were upset that family and friends were unable to understand that "it would take a while for him to catch up" or that they were unwilling to "see her as a normal child." A few mothers were pointedly critical of the conflicting messages they were getting from health professionals. For the most part, this strain stemmed from disagreements about whether the child's development was "within normal limits" or was sufficiently delayed to require therapeutic intervention.

Summary

We have highlighted some of the threats and challenges that parents described in coping with their child's birth, hospitalization, and homecoming. Figure 1.1 lists the major phases of this unfolding crisis. As this figure depicts, the crisis of newborn intensive care does not begin when their baby is admitted to the hospital or end the day parents take their baby home. For some, the delivery was preceded by a difficult pregnancy. For more parents, an uneventful pregnancy set the stage for a disquieting anaylsis of the assumptions and expectations they had held before the delivery. And, for virtually all parents, the transition home introduced new coping burdens. We have not addressed here the longer term threats to parents' well-being, because the major thrust of our study is on parents' adaptation to the hospitalization and the first few months of caring for their child at home. Nonetheless, the longer term health and development of

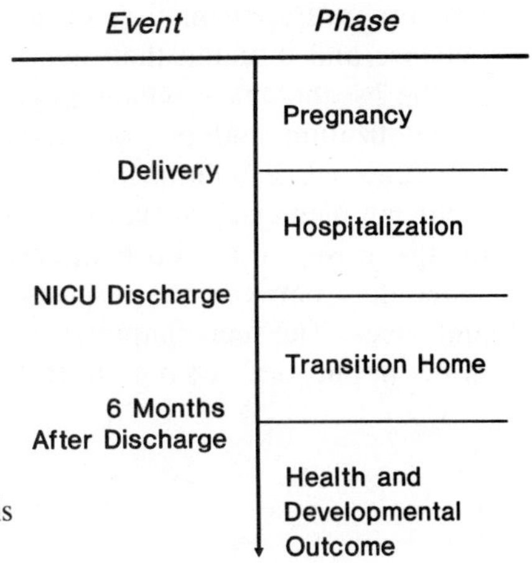

Event	Phase
	Pregnancy
Delivery	
	Hospitalization
NICU Discharge	
	Transition Home
6 Months After Discharge	
	Health and Developmental Outcome

FIGURE 1.1. Phases of the unfolding crisis of newborn intensive care.

medically fragile infants remains a concern to many parents. The uncertainty of the outcome can last for years, as we will document in the next chapter.

Were we to end our discussion here one might be left with the impression that these parents are helpless victims of a wholly traumatic experience. Fortunately, this impression would be an inaccurate one. The remainder of this book details what we learned about parents' multifaceted abilities to adapt to this unfolding crisis and about the situational and psychological factors that affected their emotional well-being and their child's developmental outcome.

Plan of the Book

In Chapter 2, we describe the background of our study, its rationale, and its procedures. In the first part of this chapter, we describe the medical setting of the NICU and review research concerning the developmental and health outcomes of children who graduate from NICUs. In the second part of Chapter 2, we describe the methods and procedures of the study.

Chapters 3 and 4 examine two ways in which parents are able to restore their assumptive world through the process of cognitive adaptation: the successful search for meaning and mastery. Chapter 5 supplies detailed findings on how mothers' beliefs about the causes of this event can aid the search for mastery and meaning. In Chapter 6, we move from an examination of cognitive adaptations to an exploration of mothers' strategies of coping with their child's hospitalization, their determinants, and their long-term consequences. Chapter 7 extends our analysis beyond mothers' intrapersonal resources to consider how other people can enhance and threaten their adaptation. In Chapter 8, we focus attention on the psychological meaning of mothers' remembrances of their child's hospitalization and on how their earlier cognitive adaptations, coping strategies, and relationships with support providers can shape their recurring memories of that time. Chapter 9 introduces a final perspective on the crisis of newborn intensive care by examining similarities and differences between the responses of mothers and fathers and husbands and wives. The final chapter, Chapter 10, integrates the key findings and draws implications of our study for helping professionals.

2
Background and
Description of the Study

The first part of this chapter depicts the medical setting in which the infants in our study were treated. We describe the physical environment of the NICU and the roles of the physicians, nurses, and parents. The second part reviews the literature on the development of infants who are typically treated on NICUs. In the last part, we summarize the methods and procedures of our study.

The Medical Setting of the Newborn Intensive Care Unit

Approximately 5% of the babies born in this country are admitted each year to NICUs (Phibbs, Williams, & Phibbs, 1981). Some of these infants, including those whose families participated in our study, are treated in regional NICUs that provide the highest level of intenstive care—in health systems parlance, Level III care. The NICU from which our study participants were drawn is a 26-bed unit located at a university medical center and serves families who live in the northern two thirds of Connecticut and in border towns of southern Massachusetts and western New York. Half of these infants are born at the university hospital and the other half are transported by ambulance from community hospitals. This unit admits approximately 450 babies a year, two thirds of whom survive to discharge.

Bogdan et al. (1982), describing their own gradual accommodation to the novel environment of several NICUs they studied, reveal how parents too must acclimate themselves to an "unknown world":

> The newcomer to a unit is struck by the pace of activity, the long intense hours that staff works, the sophisticated technology, and the life and death struggle that is a regular part of the routine. As one spends time on these units, all of those factors, plus the awesome sight of tiny infants with a substantial portion of their bodies covered with tape, attached to respirators, oxygen dispensers, IVs, monitors, under heaters and bilirubin lights, with monitors beeping warnings of heart arrest, soon become the details of everyday life (p. 7).

11

Like the NICUs observed by Bogdan et al., the unit from which our families were recruited is a busy, bright, crowded, and equipment-filled facility, designed for optimal efficiency. Parents may notice that approximately a third of the infants are on respirators at any time, a fact that reflects this unit's expertise in treating critically ill newborns. Most of the babies are in incubators that jut out from the wall, each connected to a panel of wall plugs to which many pieces of monitoring equipment are attached. These monitors, sitting on shelves above the incubators, have blinking lights and flashing numbers that provide information on heart and rspiratory functions. Periodically, monitors will emit an alarm to warn the nurse that the infant has stopped breathing or dropped his or her heart rate to a dangerous level. Some of the sicker babies, and most infants during the first hours after admission, are placed on "warmer beds": flat, open platforms with heating lights attached above to keep the infant warm. Babies lying on these beds appear much less protected and will frequently be lying in a spread-eagle position. This is often how parents see their infant for the first time after the delivery.

Parents also witness many medical emergencies when they visit the unit. When an infant's status changes suddenly, physicians and nurses cluster at the baby's bedside; a portable x-ray machine may be wheeled over, cardiopulmonary resuscitation may be initiated, emergency chest tubes may be inserted, or intravenous medications may be started.

Most of the babies on the unit at any time, however, have "settled in." Some parents paste pictures of family members or siblings' drawings in their child's incubator. Sometimes, they place cassette players inside the incubator to entertain the baby with soothing music or dolls and stuffed animals to make the incubator seem more like a baby's crib. Some of the tiniest babies are dressed in dolls' colthing parents purchased in toy departments. Whereas some of the babies are well enough to be fed by bottle, others are fed by gavage, a procedure in which a small tube is passed through the mouth into the stomach, and formula or the mother's breast milk is placed in a syringe-like container connected to the upper end of the tube and allowed to move by gravity through the tube and into the stomach.

When parents arrive at the NICU to visit their baby, they are usually met by the primary nurse. Each primary nurse is responsible during her shift for taking care of her "primary" and two or three other infants. Ideally, parents come to know their child's primary nurse as someone on whom they can rely for information and for continuity of care. Although the primary nurse's responsibility is to mediate parent–professional communication, we have heard many parents object to one consequence of this arrangement—the reduction of opportunities to speak directly to their child's physicians.

Parents usually encounter several physicians during their baby's stay on the NICU, and naturally, they may be confused about the roles and responsibilities of each. Four house officers, usually pediatric residents, are primarily responsible for medical management of the babies. Overseeing the house officers is a supervisory pediatric resident in his second year of training. The next level of staffing is occupied by a neonatology fellow, who has completed his training in pediatrics and has decided to sepcialize in the care of sick newborns. Finally, there is the attending neonatologist who is accountable for the care of all of the babies on the unit. The neonatology fellow ordinarily has more opportunity to speak with parents and shares this responsibility with the attending physician. Generally, if the baby is very sick, the attending physician will have significantly more contact with family members than when the baby is doing well or not having any acute medical crises.

The third party in the baby's care is the family. Medical and nursing staff of this NICU actively encourage parents' participation in their child's care, suggesting to parents that they touch and stroke their baby, and talk to their baby no matter how ill or unstable he might be. Some parents become very active participants, aiding where possible in medical care. Others are comfortable with gradually assuming only basic caretaking activities, such as feeding and bathing. Still others need a long time before they are able to take an active role in any aspect of caring for their baby.

Although this book focuses in part on the stresses that parents encounter in the NICU, we must not forget that NICU nurses and physicians also work in a highly stressful environment. Nurses in particular appear to suffer a high incidence of "burnout," resulting in a frequent turnover in NICU nursing staff (Marshall & Kasman, 1980). Newborn intensive care unit nurses who participated in a study by Gribbins and Marshall (1984) identified several sources of stress in meeting their professional roles and responsibilities. These included frustrations about understaffing, doubts about their professional competence, concerns about the quality of life of newborns who received aggressive treatment despite their poor prognosis, and conflicts with house officers. Such problems cannot help but interfere with nurses' efforts to comfort and assist parents.

Bogdan et al.'s (1982) study of NICU nurses' perceptions of parents merits special attention here because it reveals that nursing staff formulate implicit "theories" about effective parental adjustment to this crisis. Participants in this study distinguished well-adjusted from poorly adjusted parents according to the following criteria: The "good" parents ask appropriate questions, acknowledge the seriousness of the condition, and tolerate the uncertainty of the final outcome. They appear grateful for their baby's care and conform to the unit's policies and schedules. They visit regularly, call on the telephone, and react appropriately to both good and bad news about their baby's condition. Finally, they "bond" to their child and exhibit the potential for providing good care after discharge. The "poor" parents are unable, or refuse, to appreciate the seriousness of the problem, ask inappropriate questions, and rarely visit or call the unit.

When they do visit, it is briefly, and they appear reluctant to touch the baby. They are also seen as having few psychological or social resources to meet their baby's needs after discharge. The study's authors cautioned that these assumptions about successful and unsuccessful adjustment to newborn intensive care appear based on limited information, guided mainly by "short observations," "limited conversations," and "second-hand reporting." They suspected that few of the nurses knew what parents were really thinking or feeling and knew little about their lives outside of the hospital setting. We hope that this book will fill this gap by chronicling the crisis of newborn intensive care from the parents' perspective.

The Health and Development of Newborn Intensive Care Unit Graduates

The vast majority of graduates of intensive care units, especially those who have no medical problems other than prematurity, will develop normally and have healthy childhoods. Nonetheless, these infants as a group are at greater than average risk for developmental disabilities and chronic health problems from perinatal complications such as very low birthweight, intrauterine growth retardation, respiratory distress, seizures, asphyxia, and infections (Kopp & Kaler, 1989). Recent advances in neonatal medicine have been responsible both for improvements in the long-term health and development of those children with less severe early medical problems and the survival of those with more life-threatening conditions, now including newborns with birthweights below 1,000 g (McCormick, 1989). These new survivors, however, are especially vulnerable to severe cognitive and neurological disorders (How, Bill, & Sikes, 1988).

Problems exhibited more often by medically fragile infants during the first year include delayed acquisition of fine and gross motor skills and neuromotor abonormalities—asymmetries in motor coordination and muscle hypotonia or hypertonia (Greenberg & Crnic, 1988; Klein, Hack, Gallagher, & Fanaroff, 1985; Pederson, Evans, Chance, Bento, & Fox, 1988; Ross, Schechner, & Frayer, 1982). For some infants, these problems are transient; for others, they forecast menal retardation, physical handicaps, or learning disabilities (Ellison, 1984). Low-birthweight babies are also at higher risk of having a difficult temperament, evidenced during the first year by irritability and poor adaptability to changes in the environment (Field, Sostek, Goldberg, & Schuman, 1979; Hertzig & Mittleman, 1984). Other research shows preterm infants to be less socially responsive (Brown & Bakeman, 1980; Goldberg, 1979), to behave in ways that are more difficult to interpret (McGehee & Eckerman, 1983), and to be more difficult to feed because of their poor head control and weaker suck (Bakeman & Brown, 1980).

Longer term follow-up research on the developmental consequences of perinatal medical problems and prematurity has been largely limited to the ascertainment of major deficits in intelligence and school performance. Several recent longitudinal studies of very low birthweight infants followed to school age reveal only slight departures from normal intelligence, but a substantial incidence of "school failure" and low achievement test scores (Calame, Fawer, Claeys, Arrozola, Ducret, & Jaunin, 1986; Lefebvre, Bard, Veilleux, & Martel, 1988; Lloyd, 1984; Siegel, 1982). Twenty-five percent of one cohort of relatively healthy preterm infants who were not mentally retarded had a "learning problem" at age 8 years, as indicated by attendance in special education classes and resource rooms or retention in grade (Cohen, Parmelee, Sigman, & Beckwith, 1988). In another follow-up study of sicker premature infants, 43% encountered similarly defined school problems, and 23% were identified by school officials as learning disabled (Sell, Gaines, Gluckman, & Williams, 1985).

Ignored in these prospective studies are the more common reasons why children have difficulties in school. Numerous retrospective studies have documented a disproportionate number of premature deliveries in the histories of children with psychiatric problems (e.g., McNeil, Weirgerink, & Dozier, 1970; Zitrin, Ferber, & Cohen, 1964). Also, several prospective studies of low-birthweight infants followed into the preschool period have documented a higher than average incidence of "externalizing" behavioral disorders such as aggressiveness and hyperactivity (Raugh & Achenbach, 1987; Towle, Bach, Hauck, Katzenstein, Dweck, & Crimmins, 1987) and "internalizing" disorders such as anxiety and withdrawal (Lindgren, Harper, & Blackman, 1986). The symptoms of some of these disorders, identified in preschool-age children, do persist in some children after they enter school (Campbell, Breaux, Ewing, & Szumonowski, 1986; Palfrey, Levine, Walker, & Sullivan, 1985). Further, there is now persuasive eivdence from longitudinal studies that many children do not "outgrow" these problems but continue to encounter academic and social difficulties in adolescence and perhaps into the young adult years (Lambert, 1981). Breslau, Klein, and Allen (1988), reporting findings from a fully prospective study to school age, showed that very low-birthweight boys are significantly more likely than normal-birthweight boys to be rated by their mothers and teachers as having both externalizing and internalizing psychiatric problems.

Many graduates of NICUs also have episodic or chronic health problems that require recurrent hospitalizations, continued dependence on medical technology, and substantial ambulatory health-care services (McCormick, Stemmler, Bernbaum, & Farran, 1986). Low-birthweight infants who have continuing health problems exhibit poorer cognitive and motor development in early childhood compared to those who are healthy (Landry, Chapieski, Fletcher, & Denson, 1988). Infants whose lungs are damaged before NICU discharge (a common problem in the sample of infants in our study) are particularly vulnerable for chronic and progressive pulmonary disease (Bader, Kamos, Lew, Platzker, Stabile, & Keens, 1987; Kim, Wheeler, Logmate, & Wohl, 1988). A related concern is the impact of early and continuing medical problems on children's activities of daily living (McCormick, 1989; Stein et al., 1987). In one study (McCormick, Stemmler, Bernbaum, & Farran, 1986), 17% of preschool children who were born at low birthweights were hospitalized during the previous year, and 35% exhibited functional limitations presumably associated with continuing illness.

Although actual rates of childhood illness and utilization of health-care serices are greater in children with perinatal medical problems, the development of these children may also be influenced by parents' *perceptions* of the child's fragility. Evidence supporting this hypothesis comes from research on the "vulnerable child syndrome," a term that characterizes parents' perceptions of previously ill, but now healthy, children as frail and in need of protection (Green & Solnit, 1964). Compared to mothers of healthy-born infants, mothers of premature infants, especially infants with perinatal medical problems, tend to see their child as weaker and in greater danger of dying (DiVitto & Goldberg, 1979; Plunkett, Meisels, & Stiefel, 1986) and are more concerned about their child's appetite, risk of injury, and physical strength (Perrin, West, & Culley, 1989). Mothers who view their prematurely born youngsters as being more vulnerable for health problems may well encounter difficulty in setting age-appropriate limits, accounting for the established link between vulnerable child perceptions and behavioral problems surrounding peer relationships and self-control among preschool-age children who were prematurely born (Perrin et al., 1989).

The worrisome consequences of perinatal medical problems are acknowledged by many parents of medically fragile infants. Briggs (1985) conducted a detailed study of the emotional impact on 80 mothers who had a newborn hospitalized on an intensive care unit. Perhaps the most striking finding from this study was the high proportion of mothers who, at NICU discharge, feared for their infant's future. More than half were concerned that their child might contract a life-threatening illness and nearly as many feared that their child's development would be abnormal. Months later, these mothers continued to express anxiety about their child's development, even though three-fourths of the children had a "benign course" after discharge.

Predictive Factors

Prospective studies indicate that social factors and caregiving processes outweigh perinatal variables as predictors of later cognitive ability (Cohen & Parmelee, 1983; Siegel et al., 1982) and appear to have an even more powerful role in predicting social and cognitive outcomes among premature than among term-born infants (Greenberg & Crnic, 1988). Clearly, no single factor is sufficient to account for the variation in these children's development. Studies in which clusters of risk factors and their interactions were examined have afforded more accurate predictions of developmental outcomes for at-risk infants than those that were limited to single predictors or to the analysis of main effects (O'Grady & Metz, 1987; Rutter, 1981).

Rutter (1988) has drawn needed attention to protective factors that can interrupt the pathways from vulnerability to disorder. Werner and Smith (1982) found that infants who were at risk because of perinatal hazards and family instability enjoyed good cognitive outcomes at school age when their families received more social support. Similarly, O'Grady and Metz (1987) showed that social support moderated the effect of newborn risk indicators and stressful events on the development of childhood behavior disorders. There is substantial evidence that parents of handicapped and at-risk infants who have effective social networks are better adjusted and interact in more optimal ways with their child (e.g., Affleck, Tennen, Allen, & Gershman, 1986; Dunst & Trivette, 1987). With the exception of what has been learned about the protective effects of social support, however, little is known about why some parents adjust well and others do not and what influence these factors might have on their child's development.

Several researchers have examined differences between the adjustment of mothers of premature infants and those whose infants are born at term. Trause and Kramer (1983) compared these two groups of mothers 1 week after the delivery and several months after the baby's discharge from the hospital. In the days after the birth, mothers of premature infants described more crying, hopelessness, and concern about their ability to cope. After taking their baby home, however, there was no difference between the groups. In another comparative study of mothers in the months after hospital discharge, there were no differences in the anxiety levels of the two groups (Busch-Rossnagel, Peters, & Daly, 1984). Yet another group of investigators reported differences between these two groups in their emotional well-being during the first few days after the delivery but not months later (Jeffocate, Humphrey, & Lloyd, 1979). Together these studies indicate that initial differences between the adjustment of mothers of preterm infants and that of mothers of typical infants are short-lived and that mothers of sicker premature infants have more difficulty adjusting to newborn intensive care.

How these parents are able to adapt effectively, what determines how well they adjust, and what effects these factors might have on the development of medically fragile infants has not been the subject of systematic study. The need for this research, particularly research that is informed by theoretical paradigms of coping with stressful events, guided the design of our study.

Methods and Procedures

In this section, we describe the procedures we followed in conducting the study and the methods and instruments we used to gather information from our participants. Then, we provide a general overview of the study's prospective design and data analytic strategies. As a prologue to the multivariate data analyses of mothers' well-being and adaptation that appear in many of the chapters, we also summarize the associations among our longitudinal measures of mothers' adaptational outcomes and children's developmental outcomes. Finally, we examine the prediction of these outcomes by key background variables such as mothers' age, education, parity, and the severity of the infant's medical problems before NICU discharge.

Recruitment and Sampling

We recruited families for our study over a span of 30 months, starting in July, 1984. All of the mothers eligible for the study had a baby who was hospitalized on the NICU at the University of Connecticut Health Center in Farmington, Connecticut, a suburb of Hartford. Only those mothers whose children appeared medically stable and were to be sent home in the near future were invited to participate in the study. We devised additional criteria to narrow the pool of candidates. The mother had to be older than 16 years, be free of major psychopathology (such as major depression or substance abuse), and speak English well enough to be interviewed and to fill out our questionnaires. In addition, her baby had to have spent longer than 10 days in the NICU and have a history of at least one of a number of severe perinatal medical problems posing a high risk of subsequent health disorders, developmental disability, or both. During the recruitment phase, 157 families met these criteria and were approached to determine their interest. One hundred and fourteen, or 73%, of these mothers accepted the invitation and gave written consent to their participation in the study. The husbands of 60 of these women were also asked to take part in the study, and 50 of them agreed.

The background characteristics of the 114 families at the time they entered the study are presented in Table 2.1. These families were broadly middle class and predominantly white. The vast majority of the babies were born prematurely, at or less than 36 weeks' gestational age, and the average child spent almost 2 months on the intensive care unit.

The infants in our study received a spectrum of early intervention services in the year and a half after they were discharged from the NICU. Half of the families were randomly assigned to an experimental support program that we provided to assist parents during the first 3 months after discharge. A synopsis of the effects of this transitional support program is contained in Chapter 10, and the interested reader can consult a recently

TABLE 2.1. Descriptive statistics for the sample at NICU discharge.

Variable	Percentage	Mean	SD[a]
Mothers' age		27.76	5.08
Mothers' education (yrs)		13.54	2.06
Duration of intensive care (wks)		7.52	5.47
Birthweight (kgs)		1.52	.87
Gestational age at birth (wks)		30.75	4.47
Days on ventilator		3.08	3.59
First-born child	54.4		
Male/female child	50.0/50.0		
Two-parent family	88.6		
Caucasian family	85.8		
Perinatal complications			
Birthweight under 1500	66.7		
Intrauterine growth retardation	9.6		
Seizures	4.4		
Bronchopulmonary dysplasia	39.5		
Hydrocephalus	4.4		
Severe apnea	62.3		
Severe asphyxia	27.2		
Severe intraventricular hemorrhage	5.3		
Marked hypotonia/hypertonia	5.3		
Severe hyperbilirubinemia	12.3		
Persistent fetal circulation	12.3		

[a] Standard deviation.

published article for a fuller description (Affleck, Tennen, Rowe, Roscher, & Walker, 1989). Thirty-five percent of the children received habilitative and early educational services from state and community agencies in the first 6 months after discharge. Most in this group were enrolled in home-based early intervention programs that emphasized developmental stimulation, physical therapy, or both. In the year following, 51% of the children participated in either home-based or center-based intervention programs for children with special needs.

Data-Gathering Procedures

Before the child was discharged from the hospital, each mother and participating father was interviewed separately by a member of the research team. Most of the interviews, which were recorded on audiotape, took place in the family's home, but some, at the parents' request, were done in the hospital. The predischarge interviews were conducted by a woman who had previously been a staff nurse on this NICU. Parents also completed a battery of questionnaires at this time. Six months after NICU discharge, 104 of the mothers were visited in their homes by another interviewer, a woman with a Master's degree in counseling. They were interviewed once again and completed another set of questionnaires.

Eighteen months after NICU discharge, 94 families supplied additional information, and the child's development was assessed either in the home or at the hospital by a licensed pediatric clinical psychologist.

TOPICS COVERED IN THE INTERVIEWS

The selection of topics covered in the interviews at hospital discharge and at the 6-month and 18-month follow-ups was guided by theory and research on coping with stressful life events. The interviews themselves contained a mix of semistructured, open-ended questions and fixed-response questions commonly accompanied by rating scales. Replies to the open-ended questions were categorized by two independent judges, who demonstrated adequate interjudge reliabilities for all of the results that we present. The specific questions and coding categories are described in the chapters that follow.

Each interview at NICU discharge began with an invitation to describe, in whatever ways the parent wished, the crisis of newborn intensive care. They were also asked about the specific aspects of the crisis they personally found to be most distressing or challenging. Then, the inteviewer asked a series of questions that were organized within seven major topic areas. The first concerned parents' beliefs about the causes of their infant's medical problems, including the premature delivery. A second set of questions examined parents' appraisals of their past and future risk of pregnancy and delivery complications, their past and future prevention efforts, and their future childbearing plans. A third series of questions elicited parents' social comparisons—how they compared their baby and themselves to other sick newborns and their parents. A fourth area of questioning concerned parents' perceptions of control over their infant's recovery, treatment, and future health and development, their expectations about their child's outcome, and concerns they had about their infant's future. A fifth category included questions about the meaning of the crisis and the ways in which parents attempted to cope. A sixth section of the interview included several questions on the social support parents received during their child's hospital stay. We closed the interview by asking married parents to discuss similarities and differences between their own and their spouse's coping and the impact of any differences on their own coping and the marital relationship.

The interview with mothers 6 months after they brought their baby home from the hospital began, again, with a global question about experiences and reactions to the transition home and a specific question about the most difficult or challenging problems they were encountering. Questions were then posed in three categories. The first set of questions were directed at mothers' satisfaction with their child's outcomes and their perceived control over these outcomes. A second area of questioning pertained to mothers' future childbearing plans and the factors implicated in their decision to attempt another pregnancy. The last category of interview questions explored mother's recurring memories and emotional responses to reminders of their child's hospitalizations. These last questions were also posed to mothers at the 18-month follow-up interview.

VARIABLES MEASURED BY QUESTIONNAIRE

Parents' Strategies of Coping with Newborn Intensive Care

Mothers' and fathers' deliberate efforts to cope with their child's hospitalization were measured at NICU discharge by the Ways of Coping Checklist (Lazarus & Folkman, 1984). This checklist is designed to measure cognitive and behavioral efforts to reduce the aversiveness of a threatening experience. The scale itself lists 66 separate coping responses, each of which is rated on four-point scales reflecting its frequency of use. The scoring procedure we adopted yielded scores for five types of coping strategies: taking instrumental actions, mobilizing social support, escaping the problem, minimizing the situation, and seeking meaning in the crisis. Tennen and Herzberger (1985a) reviewed evidence of the reliability and validity of this instrument. Further details about the checklist's theoretical underpinnings and use in the stress and coping literature are given in chapter 6, where we describe mothers' coping strategies.

Intrusive Thoughts and Avoidant Responses

In chapter 8, we discuss mothers' remembrances of their child's hospilalization on the NICU, and describe their tendency to experience intrusive memories of that time and to avoid reminders of the hospitalization. At both 6 and 18 months, mothers completed the Impact of Event Scale (Horowitz, Wilner, & Alvarez, 1979). This scale was designed originally to study central features of post-traumatic stress disorder, but it has been used successfully with the much larger proportion of victims of stressful life events who do not have psychiatric disorders. This 15-item questionnaire assesses by self-report both intrusion (e.g., unbidden thoughts or images of the stressful event) and aviodance (e.g., turning away from reminders of the event, blunted sensations about the event). Mothers recorded the frequency of each response during the past week on 4-point scales. Tennen and Herzberger (1985b) review abundant evidence of the reliability and validity of this scale.

Social Support

Mothers and fathers completed a questionnaire version of the Arizona Social Support Interview Schedule (Barrera, 1981) at discharge and mothers did so once again 6 months later. Their satisfaction with, and need for, emotional, informational, and tangible support were measured on 3-point scales. At discharge, parents also completed two checklists that we developed for this study. The first elicited their satisfaction with support provided by key individuals in their social network—relatives, friends, and health-care providers. The second requested their evaluation of the support functions filled by the person they identified as the primary helpgiver. At 6 months, mothers also completed the 40-item Inventory of Socially Supportive Behaviors (Barrera, 1981) to supply a measure of the amount of support mothers had obtained in the past month. This scale measures how often others assisted mothers in managing their emotional distress, provided information and adivce, and gave material aid. Mothers' feelings of social isolation were measured by their responses to the 11-item Social Isolation subscale of the Parenting Stess Index (Abidin, 1983). Additional information on these social support scales is summarized in Chapter 7.

Adaptational Outcomes

Questionnaire assessments of parents' emotional well-being were conducted at all three waves of data collection. Mothers completed the Profile of Mood States-B (Lorr & McNair, 1982) at each wave, and the fathers completed it at NICU discharge and 18 months later. This questionnaire is a 72-item checklist of recent mood and measures six types of emotions, each on a continuum: elation/depression, composure/anxiety, certainty/ uncertainty, clearheadedness/confusion, energy/fatigue, and agreeable-ness/hostility. The score used in our analyses reflected mothers' overall mood, with higher scores representing more positive mood. In our previous studies of mothers of medically fragile infants, we have documented substantial evidence of this instrument's concurrent and predictive validity (e.g., Affleck, Allen, McGrade, & McQueeney, 1982a, 1982b; Affleck, Allen, McGrade, & McQueeney, 1983; Allen, McGrade, Affleck, & McQueeney, 1982).

Eighteen months after NICU discharge, mothers and fathers also completed the SCL-90R, a 90-item self-report inventory of psychological symptoms (Derogatis, 1977). A summary of the validity, reliability, and extensive application of this instrument is available in a review by Tennen, Affleck, and Herzberger (1985). It assesses symptoms of somatization, obsessive-compulsive behavior, interpersonal sensitivity, depression, anxiety, phobic anxiety, psychoticism, paranoid ideation, and hostility. The global index of psychological distress (Global Severity Index) was calculated and incorporated into our data analyses.

Three additional adaptational outcome variables 6 months after discharge were derived from mothers' responses to subscales of the Parenting Stress Index (Abidin, 1983). The first was the 9-item Parent Depression subscale, which assesses aspects of depression other than those tapped by the Profile of Mood States assessment of depressed mood (e.g., feelings of guilt and hopelessness). The second was the 7-item Parent Attachment subscale, which assesses emotional closeness to the child and the ability to understand the child's feelings and needs. The third was the 13-item Sense of Competence subscale, which measures the preceived degree of competence in fulfilling the parental caregiving role. Higher scores represented more optimal adpatations. Information about the reliability and validity of this instrument is available in a review and critique by McKinney and Peterson (1984).

The last two adaptational outcome variables were derived from the Home Observation for the Measurement of the Environment Inventory (HOME: Caldwell & Bradley, 1984). This 45-item scale, completed by an observer in the home, is designed to assess the quality of a young child's home environment and how much it provides opportunities for social, cognitive, and emotional development. Six subscales are scored from extensive instructions included in the manual. These are: Emotional and Verbal Responsivity of the Parent (11 items), Acceptance of the Child's Behavior (8 items), Organization of the Physical and Temporal Environment (6 items), Provision of Appropriate Play Materials (9 items), Parent Involvement with the Child (6 items), and Opportunities for Variety in Daily Stimulation (5 items). There is extensive evidence supporting the reliability and validity of this instrument as a measure of supportive environments for both typical and atypical infants and young children (Procidano, 1985). One subscale of the HOME—Mothers' Emotional and Verbal Responsivity—was rated by the interviewer based on observations she made during the home visit 6 months after discharge. The entire inventory was scored after home visits made at the 18-month follow-up. On 15 of the visits made at each wave, a second observer made independent ratings to determine interjudge reliability. Intraclass correlations documented an acceptable level of agreement.

Measurement of Infants' Characteristics

Two sets of variables capturing the medical and developmental characteristics of the infants in this study were incorporated in our data analyses. The first was an index of the severity of the child's medical problems before NICU discharge. The suitability of a composite medical severity measure was evaluated by a principal components analysis. Length of hospital stay, gestational age at birth, birthweight, amount of time on a ventilator, and the number of perinatal complications each loaded higher than .40 on a single factor that explained 80% of the variance in these measures. Accordingly, these five variables were standardized and summed to create a medical severity composite.

Eighteen months after hospital discharge, the infant's mental development was assessed with the Bayley Scales of Infant Development (Bayley, 1969), the most widely used test of an infant's developmental progress. The only departure from the usual scoring procedure was that the infant's corrected age (chronological age minus number of weeks premature) was used to calculate the Mental Development Index (MDI) from population norms. This provides a fairer comparison of these children's developmental progress with the population on which the scale was standardized. The mean MDI score for the sample was 103.7 (SD = 18.6), indicating that as a group, these children were not lagging behind their agemates' development when their age was corrected for the extent of their prematurity. Thirteen percent of the children were exhibiting a significant delay in their mental development; that is, they had scores less than 80.

To supplement this assessment of children's development, mothers were interviewed about their child's age-appropriate achievement of adaptive behavior. This was accomplished with the Vineland Adaptive Behavior Scale (Sparrow, Balla, & Cicchetti, 1984), which supplies population norms for children's communication skills, daily living skills, socialization, and motor skills and an overall adaptive behavior composite. The adaptive behavior age equivalent was divided by the child's corrected age and multiplied by 100 to yield an adaptive behavior index. The mean score was 96.33 (SD = 15.87). Seventeen percent of the children were classified as developmentally delayed in their adaptive behavior. Owing to the moderately high correlation between mental development and adaptive behavior indices ($r = .73$, $p < .001$), the child's average score on these two measures was incorporated as the developmental outcome variable in all data analyses.

A final indicator of the child's outcome was the presence or absence of a significant motor disability (e.g., spastic diplegia) observed by the examiner or documented by other health professionals who had recently seen the child. Sixteen percent of the children fell into this category. Overall, 20 of the 94 children assessed at 18 months could be classified as developmentally disabled, as evidenced by a composite developmental quotient below 80, a significant motor disability, or both.

SUMMARY OF PROSPECTIVE DESIGN AND DATA ANALYTIC STRATEGIES

Figure 2.1 lists the major categories of study variables and when they were measured. In subsequent chapters, both contemporaneous associations and predictive relations among these categories are presented and discussed. For ease of exposition, the only statistical values that are reported concern relations with parents' adaptational outcomes and the children's developmental outcomes. When other relations are described in the text, the reader can assume that they were statistically significant beyond the .05 level for two-tailed tests. We follow common analytic strategies when we consider bow cognitive adaptations, social support characteristics, and coping strategies relate to mothers' and children's outcomes. Our procedure for evaluating concurrent relations involves the construction and evaluation of hierarchical multiple regression models in which background variables (mothers' age, education, parity, and infants'

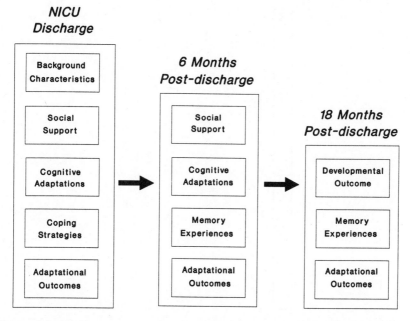

FIGURE 2.1. Major categories of study variables and their timing of measurement.

medical severity) are entered first in the equations predicting these outcomes. In some instances, the specific prediction afforded by a variable is also evaluated by controlling for its relation to mothers' well-being at the time the variable was measured. For example, the predictive significance of mothers' strategies of coping with their child's hospitalization for their well-being 18 months later is evaluated by controlling not only for background variables but also for their mood at the time they described these strategies. This conservative statistical approach helps to draw stronger inferences that certain coping strategies might improve or impede emotional adaptation. Finally, for some predictive analyses, we were interested in whether the role of early appraisals and coping responses in mothers' long-term adaptation might differ for mothers whose children develop normally or become developmentally disabled. In these instances, regression models also incorporate the child's outcome as a term in the predictive equation as well as multiplicative interaction terms capturing the effect of the predictive variable of interest that is conditional upon the child's outcome. When interaction terms are statistically significant, they are portrayed in figures to enable the reader to grasp the nature of the interaction.

TABLE 2.2. Intercorrelations among mothers' adaptational outcomes.

Variable	(1)	(2)	(3)	(4)	(5)	(6)	(7)	(8)
At NICU discharge								
(1) Positive mood								
At 6 mos.								
(2) Positive mood	.52**							
(3) Depression	−.38**	−.51**						
(4) Perceived attachment	.18	.24*	−.63**					
(5) Sense of competence	.31**	.49**	−.62**	.61**				
(6) Responsiveness	−.13	.02	−.16	.24*	.06			
At 18 mos.								
(7) Positive mood	.43**	.55**	−.34**	.29**	.34**	.09		
(8) Global distress	−.35**	−.43**	.34**	−.25*	−.21*	−.18	−.61**	
(9) Home environment	.05	.24*	−.19	.19	.08	.16	.08	−.22*

* p < .05, 92 df.
** p < .01, 92 df.

Interrelations Among Background Variables and Mothers' and Children's Outcomes

Our analyses incorporate one assessment of children's development at 18 months and nine assessments of mothers' adaptational outcomes across the 18 months of the study: mothers' mood at discharge, 6 months, and 18 months; mothers' depression, perceived attachment, sense of competence, and responsiveness at 6 months; mothers' global distress and quality of the home environment at 18 months. In this section we briefly summarize the interrelations among these outcome variables, both concurrently and over time, and the effects of background variables on these outcomes.

Table 2.2 presents the correlation coefficients calculated among mothers' adaptational outcomes. Of the 36 correlations, 22 were statistically significant. As expected, our repeated measures of emotional well-being, including mothers' reported mood, depression, and global distress, were all significantly correlated. Mood was assessed on all three occasions, and there was a moderate degree of stability in mothers' ordering on this variable over time. The observationally derived variables of mothers' responsiveness and the home environment did not relate as highly to well-being variables as the well-being variables did among themselves. For example, mothers' responsiveness 6 months did not co-vary with their mood, and the correlation between global distress and home environment was significant but low. The only significant relation between children's development at 18 months and mothers' adaptational outcomes was between less optimal home environments and lower developmental quotients ($r = -.39, p < .001$).

Table 2.3 presents the correlations between the four background

TABLE 2.3. Relations of background characteristics to mothers' adaptational outcomes.

Variable	Mothers' age	Mothers' education	Parity	Medical severity
At NICU discharge				
Positive mood	.01	.02	-.06	-.05
At 6 mos.				
Positive mood	.22*	.05	-.05	-.10
Depression	-.23*	.15	.21*	.22*
Perceived attachment	.05	.03	-.10	-.18
Sense of competence	.12	.09	-.11	-.13
Responsiveness	.07	.18	.10	-.17
At 18 mos.				
Positive mood	.12	-.12	.05	-.08
Global distress	-.09	-.02	-.07	.07
Home environment	.29**	.32**	.08	-.24*

* $p < .05$, 92 df.
** $p < .01$, 92 df.

variables and mothers' adaptational outcomes. Older mothers reported more positive mood at 6 months, less depression at 6 months, and provided more optimal home environments at 18 months. The home environments of mothers having more education were also more optimal. Mothers of first-born children reported more depression, as did mothers whose children had more severe perinatal medical problems. Mothers of more severely impaired newborns also lived in homes that were rated lower on the HOME Inventory. The only background variable that predicted infants' developmental outcomes was parity; in this sample, first-born children exhibited better developmental outcomes than later-born children. The inability of the medical severity composite (and its components) to predict developmental outcome is consistent with a number of other studies of prematurely born infants (e.g., Beckwith & Cohen, 1984; Escalona, 1982; Greenberg & Crnic, 1988).

3
The Search for Meaning

Few fail to appreciate the more obvious psychological challenges facing the parents of medically fragile infants. Any parent can imagine a mother's distress at giving birth to a premature baby, her anxiety in helplessly watching the baby struggle to survive on an intensive care unit, or her frustration in trying unsuccessfully to feed or calm her baby. Less apparent to observers is the psychological toll of feeling "victimized" by the birth and care of a medically fragile infant. Taylor, Wood, and Lichtman (1983) define a victim as "one who is harmed by or made to suffer from an act, circumstances, agency, or condition." Stripped of its adverse connotation, this definition of victimization applies to most individuals who encounter negative life events. But the very status of being a victim is neither socially nor psychologically neutral in our culture. Many undesirable social and personal consequences, beyond the obvious losses associated with the event, ensue from the experience of victimization. Negative personal consequences include the loss of control and threats to self-esteem. Negative social consequences include being blamed by others for the event, feeling stigmatized because of it, and being pitied for it.

Fortunately, individuals have a formidable capacity to reshape the meaning of threatening events, and by so doing, can minimize their status as victims. In this chapter, we show how certain beliefs about the meaning and significance of the crisis of newborn intensive care not only help parents mitigate feelings of victimization but may even foster a sense of purpose and privilege. Our discussion emphasizes three cognitive adaptations: finding a sense of order and purpose in their infant's intensive care, construing benefits or gains from this crisis, and making downward comparisons. These cognitive strategies, which Taylor et al. (1983) term "selective evaluations" of victimization can also help parents to restore some of the valued assumptions that, as was shown in Chapter 1, may be shattered by the birth of a medically fragile newborn.

Order and Purpose

The search for meaning in a threatening experience involves a wish to understand how this event fits in a world that has both order and purpose (Thompson & Janigian, 1988). People's ability to find order and purpose in adversity can be discerned in their answers to the question "Why me? Why was I the one who suffered this misfortune?" The search for an answer to this question needs to be distinguished from attempts to answer the question, "What is the *cause* of this event?", which we examine in Chapter 5. Satisfying answers to these two questions are not necessarily the same. Neither does the ability to find a cause imply that the event will be seen as a meaningful one.

To illustrate this point, consider individuals who are seriously ill with heart disease. They may well understand the possible casues of their illnes but are still searching for the reasons why they are the ones who became ill. In other words, they are trying to understand the illness' *selective* incidence (Janoff-Bulman & Frieze, 1983). Some causal ascriptions for a serious illness, for example, the belief that engaging in certain behaviors increased one's risk for the disease, may also help explain the illness' selective incidence, but many causal attributions do not help answer the question "Why me?" As one mother in our study confessed before we had even introduced this topic in the interview:

> We know that 7 out of every 100 babies are born prematurely. We know that problems with my uterus were the cause of the premature delivery. But that still doesn't answer the question, "Why us? and not someone else?".

We and other investigators have asked people who have encountered any of a number of threatening events whether they have ever asked themselves "Why me?", and if so, how they might have answered the question. Particpants in these studies include mothers of diabetic children (Affleck, Allen, Tennen, McGrade, & Ratzan, 1985), individuals with severe arthritis (Affleck, Pfeiffer, Tennen & Fifield, 1987; Lowery, Jacobsen, & Murphy, 1983), individuals who have lost their sense of smell (Tennen, Affleck, & Mendola, in press), victims of severe burns (Kiecolt-Glaser & Williams, 1987), cancer patients (Gotay, 1985); incest victims (Silver, Boon, & Stones, 1983), women with impaired fertility (Mendola, Tennen, Affleck, McCann, & Fitzgerald, in press), people with spinal cord injuries (Bulman & Wortman, 1977), parents of stillborn children (DeFrain, 1986), and mothers of babies who died unexpectedly (Wortman & Silver, 1987).

These studies demonstrate that most, but not all, of these individuals have asked the question "Why me?". Thus, the search for clues to the selective incidence of misfortune is a common, but not universal, response. The proportion of individuals who claim to have any answer to this question also varies considerably from study to study. Thus, there may be something about differences among these events that eases or hinders the search for an answer. These studies reveal that people's answers to "Why me?" comprise several categories. Some of their answers, for example, "it was just fate that something like this should happen to me" or "it was just a random occurrence," convey a sense of order (even in the random distribution of misfortune), but not a purpose. Other answers, as in unelaborated references to "God's will," suggest an underlying reason of which the person is unaware. Another common conclusion is the belief that the misfortune has a valued purpose, as in "making me more aware of the important things in life," "testing my faith in God," and (as in the case of impaired fertility) "being chosen to give love to an adopted child." Occasionally, the event is interpreted as punishment for past misdeeds or transgressions.

At hospital discharge, we asked parents the following question: "Some parents of premature or sick newborns might find themselves asking the question, 'Why me? Why was I the one who is a parent of a premature or sick newborn?'. Other parents might not find themselves asking this question. Have you ever asked the question 'Why me?'? If so, have you found any answer to this question?"

Approximately three fourths of the mothers stated that they had asked themselves the question "Why me?", and 42% said they came up with some answer. Only 10% of the mothers were satisfied to view this occurrence as a random event, a matter of chance. For them, the question, "Why me?", no longer had any meaning:

> I guess in the end that my answer to this question is "Why not me?". These things happen to people without any rhyme or reason. It was a one in a million thing, and I just happened to be that one.

> It's just something that happened. I don't blame anyone or anything. There's nothing I or anyone else could have done.

Only about 5% of the mothers made references to "fate":

> I've always thought that I'm just an accident waiting to happen. I've had a lot of bad luck in my life. All the while I was pregnant I had this feeling that something like this was going to happen.

The largest category of answers, offered by approximately 25% of the mothers, alluded to God's will or plan. A few of the mothers in this category were unable to elaborate. More viewed this as a test of faith or that they were "selected" to be the parent of a sick or premature baby. It is these mothers who apparently were able to find some specific meaning and purpose in thier plight:

> I think that this is a big test God is giving us to strengthen our faith.

> This is God's way of preparing us for the hard things that will happen in the future. If God wants to teach you something, He will cause you to experience these things to turn your head.

If a child like mine had to be born, it's a good thing that I'm his mother. I think I can really make a difference in his life. God forbid that he might have been born to someone who couldn't deal with this and would give him up for adoption.

Only two mothers thought that this event was in some way a punishment for past misdeeds. One mother mentioned her guilt over having an abortion and was distraught by this perception. But the other was able to find some valued purpose even in her punishment:

I think this is payback for some of the pain I have caused other people. I guess I'll just have to take greater responsibility for my actions and try of offset some of the harm I've done.

Our interview procedure did not allow us to distinguish between mothers who had not asked themselves the question "Why me?" because they were disinclined to search for a reason or purpose and others who had not done so because the reason or purpose was readily apparent to them. Thus, we also presented mothers with a list of statements appearing in Table 3.1. As this table shows, one fourth of these parents thought that there was no purpose or reason for this occurrence, and approximately the same proportion stated that they had never searched for a reason of purpose, or that trying to understand its reason or purpose was unimportant. Roughly half the mothers agreed with at least some of the statments endorsing a reason or purpose, particularly those statements refering to God's will or plan for them. These included the belief that they were selected by God to give care to this special baby, that this was one of the most important things that God would ever ask of them, and that this event was designed to be a test of their faith. Many of the parents who endorsed these statments had, in their answer to our open-ended question, stated that they had not asked the "Why me?" question; thus, it appears that for some, the ability to find a purpose or reason even mitigated the need to ask themselves this question.

Were certain mothers unable to find a reason or purpose? We examined

TABLE 3.1. Percentages of mothers agreeing with statements concerning reasons or purposes.

Statement	Percent
This happened because we're better able than most parents to care for a sick baby	14.6
God selected me to care for this special baby	54.8
God chooses parents who can handle a situation like this	30.8
This is probably one of the most important things of God will ask of me	52.9
This happened so that I could learn something important about myself	34.7
This situation is a test of my faith	45.2
I wonder if this is punishment for something I've done	14.6
There's no purpose or reason at all why this should have happened to us	25.0
Trying to understand why this happened isn't important to me	25.9
I have never searched for a reason or a purpose why this happened	21.1

mothers' age, educational level, parity, and the severity of the infant's medical condition as correlates of this belief and found that mothers with more education were more likely to agree that there was no purpose or reason for this event.

The inability to find a purpose or reason in this misfortune was unrelated to mother's mood reported at NICU discharge. The adaptational variables we measured 6 months after discharge—mothers' mood, depression, sense of competence, perceived attachment, and responsiveness to the child— were also unrelated to this belief, with the exception of the observational measure of mothers' responsiveness. Controlling for background variables and mothers' mood at discharge, mothers who had not found a purpose or reason exhibited less reponsiveness to their baby after discharge. These mothers did not differ on our 18-month measures of mood, global distress, and home environments, nor were there differences in their child's developmental outcome at 18 months. Thus, we have little evidence that mothers who were unable to find a reason or purpose for this event were adapting less well to intensive care and its aftermath. As we show in the next section, another cognitive adaptation—the ability to find benefits and gains in the crisis, which was unrelated to the ability to find a purpose or reason—did play a prominent role in mothers' and children's outcomes.

Benefits and Gains

Reappraising a threatening experience as beneficial or gainful is a second way in which people bring meaning to their misforture (Janoff-Bulman & Frieze, 1983; Taylor, 1983; Thompson, 1985). This cognitive adaptation gets at the heart of the event's significance for one's life goals and plans (Thompson & Janigian, 1988). If the event can be redefined in a favorable way, it loses much of its harshness. Even more, victims may thus come to see themselves as better off than they were before the event occurred.

We and other researchers have documented the benefits that victims of many types of aversive experiences attach to their misfortune. This research has included, among others, mothers of diabetic children (Affleck et al., 1985), victims of heart attacks (Affleck, Tennen, Croog, & Levine, 1987a), women with breast cancer (Taylor, Lichtman, & Wood, 1984), victims of spinal cord injuries (Bulman & Wortman, 1977) and smell disorders (Tennen et al., in press), individuals with rheumatoid arthritis (Affleck, Pfeiffer, Tennen, & Fifield , 1988), women with impaired fertility (Mendola et al., in press), people who lost their belongings in a fire (Thompson, 1985), and parents who lost a baby at birth (DeFrain, 1986). Several perceived benefits cut across these experiences. One common theme is that the event strengthened family relationshps. Another is that the experience led to positive personality changes, for example, greater patience, tolerance, empathy, and courage. Yet another common appraisal is that the experience engendered valued changes in priorities or in the ability to see what is truly important in life.

The importance of construing benefits from a threatening event was revealed most dramatically in our study of a large group of men who were followed for 8 years after suffering their first heart attack (Affleck et al., 1987a). Half of these men, 7 weeks after their attack, derived certain benefits from their misfortune, such as improved family relationships and valued changes in one's priorities. These men were significantly less likely to have a second attack over the 8 years they were followed. This relation was not confounded by social class variables or, more important, by the severity of the first heart attack. Thus, the ability to construe gains from a personal catastrophe may not only lessen distress but in certain instances may have beneficial consequences for physical health and well-being.

We have implied that it is the perception of benefits—the appraisal itself—that helps people adapt to victimization. Yet, when individuals identify greater family harmony as an unexpected benefit of a crisis, might any consequences for their well-being simply be due to their improved ability to obtain social support? If so, then this so-called "cognitive adapation" may be just an epiphenomenon, of interest only as a marker of an influential change that has occured. This is a complicated question that has yet to be addressed empirically. Our working hypothesis is that the accuracy of the benefits construed by victims is a less critical factor in adaptation than their belief that valued changes have occured. We assume that when individuals construe a beneficial change, true or not, they create a reality to which they then respond.

We explored the perceived benefits of newborn intensive care by asking mothers the following question at hospital discharge: "Some parents may see this situation as nothing but a nightmare...they can't see anything good coming out of it. Others may have found some benefits from this situation. As difficult as this situation has been for you and your family, do you see any benefits, any gains or advantages that have come from having a baby who had to be hospitalized on a newborn intensive care unit?"

Eighty percent of the mothers answered this question by describing at least one type of benefit from weathering this crisis. Many mothers said that this experience had brought them closer to their husband, other family members, and friends. For example:

> The good that came out of this was how we reacted as a couple. Something like this could tear a marriage apart if you started accusing each other. But instead, this has brought us closer together.

> Through the growth of our love for each other, I guess you could say that we've gained from this.

> We never thought we could be closer before this happened. But we did become closer. Also, I've never felt closer to my family than I have during the past month.

It was a good experience to learn who your friends really are. The ones that rallied around us are the friends I know we'll have all of our life. That's a good thing to know.

Several said that the precariousness of their child's life taught them an important lesson about keeping things in perspective:

Right after she was born, I remember having a revelation. Here she was, only a week old, and she was teaching us something—how to keep things in perspective. . .to understand what's important and what's not. I've learned that everything is tentative—you never know what life is going to bring. It's not that you stop living your day to day life, but that you come to realize that you shouldn't waste your time worrying about the little things.

This has changed my whole perspective on life. One day I was walking out of the hospital and heard two people arguing over what kind of get well card they should buy. That's so unimportant when someone's sick and maybe his life is at stake.

Some parents believed that their ability to empathize with others was enhanced:

In trying to deal with an adversity, you naturally become more sensitive to the plight of others who have gone through bad times.

A large proportion claimed positive personality changes from the personal growth that ensued from this event:

I've learned that I'm a much stronger person than I had thought. I look back, see how far I've come, and I'm very pleased in such a short period of time.

Another commonly cited benefit was the fact that their child had become more precious to them because of his or her closeness to death:

The good that's come out of this is that I marvel at what a miracle she is, what a miracle it is that she's alive and that we are going to be able to take her home.

Finally, some parents expressed gratitude for the excellent care and support extended to them and their baby in the hospital:

I'm so grateful for all of the people that helped him to live and helped me to understand. It was wonderful to learn that there are so many caring and dedicated people.

To supplement our interview question on benefits and gains, we presented mothers with a list of statements describing possible benefits or gains from this situation. These statements, and the proportions of mothers who "moderately" or "strongly" agreed with them, are listed in Table 3.2. Echoing the findings presented above, a minority of the mothers—fewer than 15%—stated that nothing good had come out of the experience. The vast majority thought that they had grown closer to their loved ones, had reassessed their priorities in a valued way, or had grown both emotionally and spiritually as a result of surviving this crisis.

TABLE 3.2. Percentages of mothers agreeing with statements concerning benefits or gains.

Statement	Percent
My baby is much more precious to me because of what we went through together	86.4
I feel much closer to my child because this happened	37.9
This experience has made me a stronger person than I was	87.4
This experience has made me look at life differently: I have a better perspective now	81.8
This experience has taught me to be grateful for the things I have in life	87.4
This experience has shown me how many people care about me	86.7
I've learned from this that I can cope with tragedies in my life	72.8
This event has brought our family members closer together	75.7
I have felt closer to my loved ones since this happened	70.9
From this, I've learned to appreciate what's important in life	84.5
My life has taken a turn for the better since this happened	31.4
This situation has brought me and my baby's father closer	70.6
This experience has renewed my faith in God	55.9
Nothing good at all has come out of this experience	12.6

Mothers who agreed more strongly with the statement that nothing good had come from this situation did not differ from the others according to their age, education, parity, or the severity of their child's medical problems. They did report less positive mood at NICU discharge ($r = -.22$, $p < .05$). They also did 6 months later, but not when their earlier mood was partialled from the correlation. The belief that nothing good had come from this situation did not predict their depression, perceived attachment, sense of competence, or responsiveness to the child 6 months later.

Although the failure to find something positive about the NICU crisis did not predict mother's adaptation 6 months later, it did predict outcomes at 18 months. Specifically, this appraisal predicted less positive mood ($r = -.33$, $p < .001$) and greater global distress ($r = .27$, $p < .01$). It also predicted lower developmental scores for the child ($r = -.37, p < .001$).

The specificity of these longitudinal relations was examined through hierarchical regression models. After entering background variables and mothers' mood at discharge, the amount of variation in 18-month outcomes predicted by this appraisal was determined. The results of these analyses show that finding no benefits in this situation was still a significant predictor of mothers' global distress and positive mood and their child's developmental outcome even when the background variables and mothers' mood at the time this appraisal was offered were taken into account.

In further analyses, we tested our hypothesis that it is the *appraisal* of benefits, more that what these statements might indicate about improved coping resources (e.g., social support), that makes a difference. Benefit statements that alluded to the strengthening of close relationship were not correlated with mother's global satisfaction with the support they obtained while their baby was hospitalized (see Chapter 7). But, mothers who cited an improved relationship with their baby's father as a benefit of this crisis were in fact more pleased with the support he provided. Whereas mothers who claimed an improved relationship with their partner scored lower on the global distress measure at 18 months ($r = -.24, p < .05$), this relation was not significant when mother's satisfaction with their partner's support was taken into account. This means that a mother who pointed to a closer marital relationship as a benefit of this crisis may well have adapted better because of the greater support she derived from this improved relationship.

Downward Comparison

A third cognitive adaptation that can bring comfort to victims of undesirable events is the comparison of their situation with worse alternatives, that is, making a downward comparison. Social comparison theory (Festinger, 1954) has long guided efforts to understand how people use social information to evaluate their skills and abilities accurately when objective indicators are lacking (Suls, 1977). More recently, it has stimulated research on how people distort, and even construct, information about others to enhance the self (Taylor & Lobel, in press; Wills, 1987). Cognitive biases in making self–other comparisons have been elucidated in a wide-ranging series of studies on the role of adaptive illusion in mental health (see Taylor & Brown, 1988 for a review) and in coping with adversity (e.g., Burgess & Holstrom, 1979; Schulz & Decker, 1985; Taylor, 1983; Thompson, 1985). This research shows that under ordinary circumstances, people tend to evaluate their personal attributes more favorably than objective evidence would warrant and that under threatening circumstances, they are apt to compare themselves with less fortunate others, both real and imagined. This proclivity of nonvictims to make unrealistically positive self–other comparisons and of victims to make "downward social comparisons' (Wills, 1981) supplies the theme of this section on the role of comparison processes in bringing meaning and comfort to parents of medically fragile infants.

Taylor and her colleagues (Taylor, 1983; Talyor & Lobel, in press; Wood, Taylor, & Lichtman, 1985) initiated formal research on social comparisons in serious illness with a study of women with breast cancer. They found a preponderance of downward comparisons in these women's appraisals of themselves and their situation. These women appeared to have searched actively for comparisons concerning their illness and their coping abilities that helped them to feel relatively advantaged. Further, those who were in the eariler phases of contending with this problem were more likely to make downward comparisons, perhaps because these comparisons freed them from "being overwhelmed by new, frightening circumstances" (Wood et al., 1985, p. 1181).

Evidence supporting the use of downward comparison as a strategy of coping with negative events is also available in studies of individuals with rheumatoid arthritis (Affleck, Tennen, Pfeiffer, Fifield, & Rowe, 1987; Affleck, Tennen, Pfeiffer, & Fifield, 1988; DeVellis et al., in press), women with impaired fertility (Affleck & Tennen, in press), and victims of fires (Thompson, 1985), rape (Burgess & Holstrom, 1979), and smell loss (Tennen et al., in press).

Elsewhere (Affleck et al., 1987), we summarized our findings on these mothers' social comparisons before their infant was discharged from the NICU. They had had extensive opportunities to compare their baby with dozens of other sick or premature babies who had been hospitalized at the same time as well to compare themselves with the other parents who could be observed or approached when they were visiting their child on the unit.

Approximately 20% of the mothers spontaneously compared their own infant to other sick infants when they were invited at the beginning of the interview to describe the crisis of newborn intensive care. We consider this a high proportion in view of range of topics that mothers were free to discuss. All to these mothers except one made downward comparisons. For several mothers, such as the two quoted next, a downward comparison appeared an immediate way of coping with their first visit to the NICU:

> The first time I saw my baby, he looked wonderful compared to some of the other babies on the unit. He was very tiny and attached to all these wires and tubes, but the other babies looked a lot worse. Their skin seemed transluscent, all full of blotches, and discolored.

> I remember standing at the door of the unit, worried to dealth about what my baby would look like. When I walked over to the isolette, I just fell apart completely. But then I looked around and saw several babies who were smaller than mine. And there was one baby whose head was bigger than his body. In a way, that helped calm me down.

Like women with breast cancer (Wood et al., 1985) and individuals with rheumatoid arthritis (Affleck, Tennen, Pfeiffer, & Fifield, 1988), these mothers compared selectively on physical dimensions of the problem that made their infant's condition seem less serious than others'. Mothers of the smallest babies, for example, tended to compare their child to those who needed more technological support to stay alive. For example:

> Things could have been a lot worse. My child wasn't on a respirator like so many others were, and she wasn't on oxygen for more than 24 hours.

Conversely, mothers of infants who were larger, but in some ways sicker, compared their infant to those who were smaller.

Fewer mothers, approximately 9%, made spontaneous comparisons to other parents of medically fragile infants. Yet all of those who did, including the parents quoted below, made downward comparisons:

Whenever I would visit the NICU, I would feel so much sympathy for some of the others. Some of them seemed so helpless, so unable to cope with all of this.

I would carefully watch how other parents would react to bad news about their baby. I must have been better informed because they seemed not to be upset by the news. If you really knew what was happening, you would have to be upset!

The latter comment is noteworthy because it reveals how a potentially demoralizing upward comparison concerning a manifest behavior can be mitigated by making a downward comparison concerning its meaning or significance. That is, the salient feature of this mother's view of herself as being more distressed that other parents was that it reflected her exceptional understanding of the threatening aspects of ths situation.

Many of our participants also volunteered that their infant's outcome was better than it could have been. Twenty-five percent of the mothers, when describing the intensive care experience, made this type of downward comparison, which lacks a specific comparison target and is labeled by Wood et al. (1985) as a *dimensional* comparison. Not surprisingly, most of these mothers compared their infant's survival to his possible death. The tone of their comments did not leave us with the impression that this was always an afterthought—an obligatory attempt to remind themselves, as others often did, that things could have been worse. In fact, several added that their child had become more precious to them simply because he had been so close to death. Some, for example, confessed their admiration for their baby's "fighting spirt" or ability to "beat the odds."

The greater prevalence of downward versus upward comparisons in mothers' descriptions of the newborn intensive care crisis paralleled ratings they made of their child's and their own comparative status. Few parents judged their infant's medical condition to be worse than average or their own adjustment as being worse than that of the avergae parent in this situation. Of course, not all infants and parents could be doing better than average. Thus, many mothers either underestimated the well-being of the averge baby or the adjustment of the average parent, or overestimated their baby's wellness or their own adjustment. In either event, a bias toward downward comparison was evidenced in their conclusions. In justifying their conclusions, mothers most often claimed that their child seemed to be larger or to need less medical intervention and that they were better able to control negative emotions and thoughts, were more informed about their child's condition and treatment, and were developing a closer attachment to the baby.

Other information gathered at NICU discharge and 6 months later extend these findings. At hospital discharge, mothers also rated how important it was for them to know how other babies and parents were doing. Parallcling our finding of more frequent social comparison state- ments about their baby than about themselves, mothers were significantly more interested in assessing the medical condition of other infants than the coping and well-being of other parents. Interestingly, those who were more interested in the medical status of other infants were more apt to make downward comparison statements about their child when they described the crisis of newborn intensive care. Thus, mothers who may have been searching more actively for social comparison information may have been more likely to derive downward comparisons from their observations.

The role of downward social comparisons in mothers' appraisals of newborn intensive care was also reflected in their later memories of their child's hospitalization. When asked 6 months after NICU discharge to describe their continuing remembrances of their child's hospitalization, many mothers revealed how the social comparisons they had made then remain part of their long-term memory of this crisis:

> I have memories of that time when I look at the pictures that we took then and begin to reflect on how small she was. And then I begin to remember all of the other babies we saw and how many of them were even smaller.

> When I find myself remembering that time, I also remember all the other babies who were so much worse off.

> It's funny, but my memories aren't so much about how my own baby was back then. Instead I seem to be remembering all of the other babies who didn't make it or who probably didn't turn out as well as mine.

> Some days when I'm watching her sleeping, I'll begin to remember what a rough time we had. I'll begin to wonder why this had to happen. And then I'll think about how some of the other babies were worse off, and how lucky I really was.

> It makes me happy to remember that time. What makes me happy is that he made it. A lot of babies didn't. I'm always thinking about this one mother whose baby was bigger but he died.

In our interview 6 months after NICU discharge, we asked these mothers once again to compare their adjustment with that of the average parent caring for a medically fragile infant. As earlier, few rated their adjustment as poorer than average. There was a significant, but low, correlation between their social comparison judgments at this time and those they had made 6 months earlier. Many of the dimensional comparisons they had cited at discharge were cited once more at 6 months. But new dimensions of downward comparison emerged and were related to the assumption of full-time care. These included their perceptions of themselves as better than average caregivers and of their ability to normalize their child's care, as in avoiding the temptation to overprotect the child.

Although we did not formally assess mothers' comparisons of their infant's condition at 6 months, several volunteered downward comparisons in the course of the follow-up interview. These were offered for the most part by mothers whose child was exhibiting developmental delays, having recurring illnesses, or was temperamentally difficult. For example, one mother of a physically handicapped child said:

> I have faced the reality that she will be physically handicapped for life. But she'll probably only need braces and crutches, not the wheelchair that other children like her sometimes need.

Another, commenting on her child's delayed motor skills, said:

> His motor skills aren't what they should be. But I'm very fortunate compared to other parents because he's such a happy baby.

Finally, a mother of a baby whose schedules of hunger and sleep were unpredictable and who was hard to soothe during frequent episodes of distress told us:

> My nephew had cancer so this all seems so trivial. At least my child is healthy and she'll live. With cancer, you never know.

Yet another source of evidence for social comparison comes from our inspection of mothers' reasons for desiring interaction with other parents of NICU-treated infants. They were asked whether and why they were or were not interested in making such contacts. Consistent with Wortman nad Dunkel-Schetter's (1979) analysis of the benefits of mutual support, most mothers wanted contact with similar others in order to reduce their feelings of isolation and to compare their situation to that of other parents. Twenty percent said that they sought such contacts in order to compare themselves to other parents, and 17% in order to compare their child to other children who were on the unit. Yet, not all mothers wanted to engage other parents in order to make such comparisons. In fact, one in five mothers said that they desired no contact with other parents *because* their situation seemed to be too unique to allow any helpful comparisons.

Correlates of Social Comparisons

At discharge, mothers made a social comparison of their baby's condition on a 3-point scale, with 1 representing mothers' opinion that their baby's condition was worse than that of the average infant on the unit and 3 representing the view that their baby's condition was better than average. This rating was unrelated to the objective severity of the condition and did not correlate with their current mood. Those who expressed more favorable comparisons about their infant's condition were less depressed 6 months after discharge ($r = -.22, p < .05$), but this relation did not hold up when background characteristics and mothers' mood at discharge were controlled. Using a similar scale, mothers who rated their comparative adjustment as better than that of the average parent did report more positive mood at discharge ($r - .23, p < .05$), but did not differ on measures made at the 6-month follow-up. Neither of the comparison ratings made before discharge predicted 18-month outcomes for mothers or children. At 6 months, mothers who viewed themselves as adjusting better than the average parent in this situation were in fact less depressed ($r = -.29, p < .01$) and expressed a greater sense of competence ($r = .31, p < .01$). This comparative self-perception did not predict outcomes assessed at 18 months. These findings converge on the conclusion that mothers who compare themselves favorably to other parents of intensive-care–treated infants may, in fact, be adjusting better to the hospitalization and the transition home.

Temporal Comparisons

To this point, we have concerned ourselves exclusively with social comparison: how parents compare their child or themselves to other real or imagined individuals. Albert (1977), Suls and Mullen (1982), and Wills (1987) drew attention to people's use of *temporal* comparisons in making self-evaluations and in coping with threatening circumstances.

We uncovered two sources of evidence for temporal comparison. First, in describing the crisis of newborn intensive care, 12% of the sample spontaneously compared their infant's survival to the occurrence of earlier reproductive disappointments that are relatively commonplace in this population, such as infertility, miscarriages, and stillbirths. For example, one mother said:

> My baby was born when I was 6 months pregnant. I was so happy and relieved that I hadn't miscarried, like I had in two earlier pregnancies. My parents and brother were so upset, but I couldn't understand why. This is no big deal compared to what I went through when I lost my other babies.

Second, downward temporal comparisons played a role in mothers' active memories of their child's intensive care (see Chapter 8 for a detailed discussion). Six months after discharge, two thirds of the mothers said that they were continuing to have memories of how sick or close to death their baby had been in the hospital. And nearly half of the mothers reporting this memory added a spontaneous downward temporal comparison concerning their child. For some mothers, such as the two quoted below, a downward temporal comparison seemed to interrupt the distress stemming from this painful memory:

> Sometimes when I'm feeding him, I'll start feeling upset because I start to remember how difficult it was to feed him in the hospital. *Then I find myself comparing that with how much he eats now, and that makes me feel better.*

> When I'm in a sad mood, I find myself picturing him so sick, seeing him with all the tubes, and remembering what awful things he had to go through. *Then I start to think of how much better he's doing now, and I start feeling happy.*

In this chapter, we have described the many ways by which mothers of medically fragile infants pursue the meaning of their child's hazardous delivery, intensive care, and any problems encountered during the transition home. Most parents were able to reappraise this threatening experience in ways that made a potentially senseless occurrence a meaningful one, or at least a less aversive experience that it might have been. Their capacity to find a purpose in the crisis, their ability to construe benefits and gains from their misfortune, and their proclivity to compare their plight with less desirable alternatives helped them to mitigate a sense of victimization and its accompanying stigmatization and threats to self-esteem. In the next chapter, we expand our discussion of cognitive adaptation to ways in which mothers were able to restore a sense of mastery in this crisis.

4
The Search for Mastery

One of the demoralizing consequences of the birth and hospitalization of a medically fragile infant is, for some parents, the loss of a sense of personal control over events. In Chapter 1, we described how the child's premature birth and intensive care upset many parents because it revealed how little control they had over their childbearing outcomes. The hospitalization itself was another arena in which some mothers expressed dismay at their inability to exercise control.

The search for mastery, like the pursuit of meaning, is a major theme in coping with threat. Taylor (1983) observes that when people face an aversive event, two of the more pressing questions they ask are, "What can I do to prevent it from happening again?", and "What can I do to manage the problem now?" In this chapter, we describe parents' efforts to restore a sense of mastery over their livers. First, we examine their appraisals of personal control over outcomes after they had occurred—their child's recovery on the NICU and health and development after discharge. In addition to these retrospective control perceptions, we examine the meaning of mothers' *expectancies* of control over future events, including their child's subsequent health and development and the outcome of future pregnancies. Finally, we highlight important individual differences in mothers' desire for personal control over their infant's medical care and treatment in the hospital and the significance of mothers' outcome expectancies regardless of their appraisals of control. Before proceeding to these findings, we provide a brief review of the literature on the benefits of perceived control.

The Benefits of Personal Control

Perceptions of personal control figure in many accounts of how people cope with threatening events (Klinger, 1975; Langer & Rodin, 1976; Miller, 1980; Rothbaum, Weisz, & Snyder, 1982; Seligman, 1975; Thompson, 1981). Personal control has been defined in several ways (e.g.,

Steiner, 1979; Thompson, 1981). We favor Burger's (1989) definition of personal control as the "perceived ability to significantly alter events" (p. 246). This definition requires only that the person *perceive* a link between personal actions and outcomes; it does not require that one actually has some control over events. In some instances, an illusion of control may be as adaptive as having actual control (Langer, 1975).

There is abundant evidence that individuals facing any of a spectrum of threatening experiences adapt better when they perceive control over the consequences of the problem or its recurrence. This includes people with a variety of illnesses (Felton & Revenson, 1984), specifically, breast cancer (Taylor et al., 1984), rheumatic diseases (Nicassio, Wallston, Callahan, Herbert, & Pincus, 1985; Westbrook, Gething, & Bradbury, 1987), and epilepsy (Glueckauf & West, 1981). Other populations in which this relation has been established include caregivers of individuals with Alzheimer's disease (Page, Becker, & Coppel, 1985) and victims of spinal cord injuries (Schultz & Decker, 1985). In an earlier study of mothers of medically fragile infants, we found that perceptions of control related to mothers' well-being shortly after their infants' discharge from the NICU (Affleck, Tennen, & Gershman, 1985; Tennen, Affleck, & Gershman, 1986).

Thompson (1981) offered three reasons why personal control can reduce the stress associated with threatening events. The first is that personal control increases the predictability of the event as it unfolds. When one believes that the event is regulated by one's own actions, one can better anticipate its consequences, good or bad. A second, related reason why personal control is advantageous is that it sets an upper limit on the adverse consequences of the event. In Thompson's (1981) view, "persons with control responses available know that the situation will not become so aversive that they connot handle it" (p. 97). A third explanation of the benefits of personal control is that undercuts the feelings of helplessness and incompetence that can stem from a traumatic event. This explanation assumes that people have a basic need to feel a sense of mastery over the environment (deCharms, 1968). Hence, any threat to this motive will itself be upsetting and may lead not only to diminished self-esteem but also to depression (Peterson & Seligman, 1984; Seligman, 1975). Taylor (1983) adds yet another explanation: the perception of control increases the likelihood that one will take actions that actually improve the outcome of the stressful event.

Retrospective Control Appraisals

We begin our analysis of mothers' ability to restore a sense of mastery by examining the ways in which they believed they had influenced their child's outcome in the hospital or during the transition home. At NICU discharge,

TABLE 4.1. Percentage of mothers describing
activities that helped to influence their infant's
recovery in the hospital.

Activity	Percent
Visiting the hospital frequently	71.1
Providing social stimulation	69.3
Providing breast milk	21.1
Caretaking activities	21.1
Supplying stimulating objects/toys	11.4
Praying/religious devotions	10.5
Monitoring the infant's health care	8.8

mothers were asked to describe any and all activities undertaken that they
judged to have had a positive influence on their infant's health and development in the hospital. In addition, they rated the extent to which their
infant's progress and recovery in the NICU was owing to things that they
had done personally (0 = "no influence whatsoever" to 10 = "extreme
influence"). The average mother's rating on the 11-point scale was 5.03
(SD = 2.72). Thus, as a group, mothers thought they had exercised a
moderate amount of personal control over their infant's recovery, but
there were also considerable individual differences in the extent of
perceived control over this outcome.

Table 4.1 presents a list of the major categories of personal control
activities and the proportions of mothers who believed that these activities
afforded them a sense of control. As these results show, the vast majority
of mothers believed that they had been able to do something that helped
their child in the hospital. In particular, many parents emphasized the
importance of their regular visiting patterns and what they were able to
accomplish during those visits:

Going to the hospital all the time and being allowed to touch him, get close to
him, and hold him was good for both the baby and me. It was a terrific confidence builder. It also gave us a lot a hope that his problems were controllable.

For a month all we could do was to touch him through the little holes in the side
of the isolette. Most of the time he would jump when I touched him, and I was
afraid that I might hurt him. But I would come everyday to visit, to feel that I
was doing something for him. Maybe it did make a difference because he seems
to know my voice and he responds to it right away.

I thought it was very important for me to supply breast milk for her. This was
something I felt I could do to help from the very beginning. I also thought it was
important for me to hold her. . .for her to feel human comfort and warmth. I
did make a big effort to spend a lot of time, just holding her and talking to her.

When we spoke to him, he'd open his eyes a little. The nurses noted that he
wouldn't do that when we weren't around. It was good to know that our touch

and our voice meant something to him. That was a good thing to happen in those dark days, because we felt a connection to him.

Retrospective Control Appraisals After Discharge

Several mothers admitted that they had been able to regain a sense of control over their child's care and outcome only after they had taken their baby home:

> I feel a lot more confident now. I really feel like his mother for the first time. Before, it was the hospital that was in control. Now it's me.

> Even though he's still having problems, I feel like I'm more in control now. In the hospital, I was just a bystander. It was the hospital's baby, not mine. It's very tiring taking care of him, but I'm enjoying the feeling of being the one who can make a difference in his life.

> I'm the one who has the say now. When she was in the hospital, it was other people who called the shots. Now it's up to me. I have the control over what happens to her.

As part of the 6-month interview, mothers were again asked to rate the degree of personal control they believed they had over their child's outcome after discharge. This time, five outcome domains were rated separately. These were the child's mental development, motor development, health status, sleep patterns, and eating habits. These ratings were made on scales of 0 = "no personal control whatsoever" to 10 = "extreme amount of control." In rank order of perceived controllability, mothers' mean ratings were 6.98 (SD = 1.97) for mental development, 6.36 (SD = 2.34) for motor development, 6.31 (SD = 2.68) for health, 5.67 (SD = 3.37) for eating, and 4.95 (SD = 3.22) for sleeping.

We examined the relations among the five perceived control ratings to judge the suitability of creating composite control variables for additional analyses. A principal components analysis identified two factors with eigenvalues greater than 1. The ratings of personal control over the child's mental development, motor development, and health loaded highly on the first factor. Ratings of control over the child's eating habits and sleeping patterns loaded highly on the second factor. Thus, mothers did not appear to perceive a global sense of control over these outcomes. Rather, they appeared to differentiate control over their child's health and development from control over their child's vegetative characteristics of eating and sleeping.

We then determined whether mothers' dissatisfaction with their child's outcome at 6 months might lead them to view these outcomes as being less subject to personal control. The graph in Figure 4.1 portrays the numbers of mothers who expressed dissatisfaction with their child's outcome in the five domains. For the three outcome domains over which mothers had perceived the greatest personal control—mental development, motor

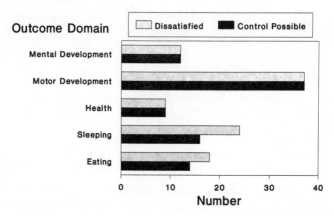

FIGURE 4.1. Numbers of mothers who were dissatisfied with their child's progress but who still believed that personal control was possible.

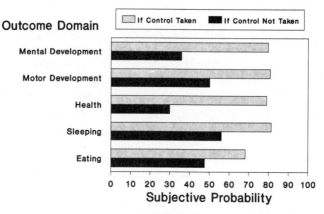

FIGURE 4.2. Subjective probability of improvement if dissatisfied mothers took control or did not take control over the outcome.

development, and health—each dissatisfied mother still believed that opportunities to exercise control were still available. But, for the two outcomes preceived as less controllable—eating and sleeping—some, but not most, of the dissatisfied mothers thought that future control was unlikely. Figure 4.2 enumerates the subjective probabilities of improvement in these outcomes for dissatisfied mothers when they imagined the effects of acting versus not acting to improve the outcome. These results parallel those presented in Figure 4.1 because the differences in anticipated improvement from taking versus not taking control were greater in the three areas over which mothers had already perceived the greatest control. Together, the patterns exhibited in these figures suggest that for the most part, mothers do not abandon their beliefs in control even even when they are displeased with their baby's progress.

Correlates of Retrospective Control Appraisals

Three variables reflecting mothers' perceived control over their child's outcome were inspected as correlates of mothers' age, education, parity, mood at discharge, severity of the infant's medical condition in the hospital, and outcome variables assessed at 6 and 18 months. The first was the global control rating made at NICU discharge. The second and third were derived from the previously described factor analysis of control ratings made at 6 months: the perception of control over the infant's mental development, motor development, and health, and the perception of control over the infant's eating and sleeping. The predischarge control rating was correlated with the 6-month rating of control over the child's health and development but not with the appraisal of control over the child's eating and sleeping.

The only significant differences in perceived control owing to mothers' and infants' characteristics at discharge were due to the severity of the infant's medical problems. Mothers of the most severely ill infants tended to perceive a greater degree of personal control over their infant's recovery in the hospital. Six months later, however, these mothers perceived *less* control over their infant's eating and sleeping.

The relation between these control appraisals and mothers' and children's outcomes measured at 6 and 18 months are presented in Table 4.2. The perception of personal control before NICU discharge was

TABLE 4.2. Correlations of mothers' retrospective control appraisals with mothers' adaptation and children's development.

Variable	Discharge control	Six mos.[a]	
		Control 1	Control 2
At 6 mos.			
Profile of mood states	.17	.21*	.31**
Depression	.07	.00	.11
Perceived attachment	−.01	.14	.13
Sense of competence	.02	.24*	−.19
Responsiveness	−.03	.20*	.18
At 18 mos.			
Profile of mood states	.05	.11	.36*
Global distress index	.12	.12	−.19
HOME inventory	−.04	.06	.21*
Developmental outcome	−.01	.12	.15

[a] Control 1 = development and health. Control 2 = eating and sleeping.
* $p < .05$.
** $p < .01$.

unrelated to these outcomes. However, each of the control appraisals at 6 months correlated at that time with mothers' positive mood and sense of competence. Mothers who perceived greater personal control over their child's health and development after NICU discharge also displayed greater responsiveness to their child during the 6-month home observation. Table 4.2 also indicates that mothers' perception of control over their child's eating and sleeping habits predicted both positive mood and higher scores on the HOME Inventory a year later. In a multiple regression equation controlling for background variables and mood at 6 months, the relation between mothers' perceived control in this area and their positive mood at 18 months remained significant.

Expectancies of Control Over Childrens' Outcome

Our findings so far suggest that mothers who have perceived a link between their own efforts and their child's outcome may have been comforted by this appraisal and may be better able to assist their child's development. It is important to distinguish these mothers' conclusion that they had controlled the outcome from their expectation that the outcome could be controlled. Several theorists argue that *expecting* control can be maladaptive when efforts to exercise that control come at great personal cost, when the expected outcome is not achieved, or when control-related activities are not carried out as anticipated (Averill, 1973; Bandura, 1977; Thompson, 1981).

At NICU discharge, mothers rated the extent to which their child's normal health and development would depend on certain things they must do (0 = not at all dependent to 10 = totally dependent; mean = 5.91, SD = 3.00). The specific activities that they believed were necessary to improve their child's future health and development are listed in Table 4.3. A large proportion of mothers anticipated the need to protect their child from potentially harmful exposures to viruses and other agents that could lead to serious respiratory problems. They foresaw having to prohibit others from smoking around the baby, to screen visitors for colds, to keep the baby

TABLE 4.3. Percentages of mothers anticipating activities that would help their child's future health and development.

Activity	Percent
Extraordinary protections	43.9
Careful monitoring of health and development	41.2
Treat child normally	18.4
Carry out recommended therapies/interventions	17.5
Extra love and affection	9.6
Extra stimulation	8.8

inside during cold weather, or avoid crowds, and so forth. Nearly as many mothers planned to monitor carefully their child's health and development, expecting frequent physical and developmental exams. Fewer spoke of the need to carry out recommended therapies, to provide extra stimulation, or to be more affectionate than would normally be required for a child to develop normally. In contrast, nearly 20% of the mothers thought that they would have to do nothing out of the ordinary to enhance their child's opportunities for a normal outcome. All that was necessary was to treat their baby as one would a "normal child."

Mothers who expected greater control over their child's outcome did not differ on background variables, nor were their child's medical problems any more or less severe. Their control expectancy did not figure in their mood at hospital discharge, nor did it predict the control they actually thought they had exercised over their child's outcome 6 months after discharge. Yet, those who had expected greater control reported less positive mood at 6 months ($r = -.23$, $p < .05$) and scored higher on the global distress measure at 18 months ($r = .29$, $p < .01$). The relation between higher control expectancies and greater distress in the second year after discharge was independent of background variables and mothers' mood at discharge.

Would the perceived "failure" to prevent a poor outcome engender even greater emotional distress in those mothers who had anticipated greater personal control over their child's development? In two equations, one predicting mothers' mood and the other predicting mothers' global distress at 18 months, background variables and mothers' mood at discharge were entered along with the presence or absence of a developmental disability at 18 months and mothers' expectancies of control. With these variables in the equation, we tested the significance of the interaction between expected control and the diagnosis of a developmental disability at 18 months. The latter term did not make a significant contribution to the prediction equation, suggesting that mothers who had expected greater control were more distressed at 18 months regardless of their child's outcome.

It appears, then, that the emotional benefits of perceiving control over the child's outcome after the fact do not extend to the expectation of control over the outcome. We suspect that many of the mothers who had anticipated greater contol were those who had made many burdensome accommodations to see this through. For these mothers, control efforts may have come at great cost to their own well-being, through personal sacrifice and alterations in family life. One mother who had expected considerable control before she took her baby home described this dilemma 6 months after discharge:

I became almost obsessed with protecting her when she came home from the hospital. I wouldn't let anyone come into the house. I wouldn't let anyone breathe on her. I was constantly disinfecting my hands. Maybe this isn't worth it, raising her in a "bubble," worrying about the slightest thing that might happen. What kind of life is this for her? What kind of life is it for me?

Alternatively, some mothers' control expectancies may not have been matched by their self-efficacy (Bandura, 1977). That is, they may have been distressed to find that the appropriate actions were not within their reach. And, despite the finding that the long-term consequences of mothers' control expectancies were unaffected by the diagnosis of developmental disability, these mothers may have been more disappointed by even minor problems in their child's development, viewing them as instances of personal failure. As one mother lamented:

> The hardest part is realizing that this person is totally dependent on me for whatever his future brings. This has put tremendous pressure on me to do the right things. But I'm very upset that I haven't been getting much in return, that there's been very little response to my best efforts.

Our findings echo those reported by Lyman, Wurtele, and Wilson (1985) in a study of mothers of premature infants who went home on apnea monitors. Mothers in their study who had higher expectations of control in this situation were more anxious than mothers who had lower control expectancies. Apparently, feeling responsible for their child's survival increased these parents' distress.

Expectancies of Control Over Future Pregnancies

Another area in which we studied mothers' control expectancies was control over the outcome of future pregnancies. Unlike the foregoing analysis of childrens' outcome, we are unable to judge the significance of pregnancy control expectancies after the outcome of future pregnancies is known because few mothers had additional children during our 18-month follow-up.

At NICU discharge, we asked mothers to rate, on a 0 to 10 scale, how much personal control they believe they had over preventing a recurrence of newborn intensive care should they become pregnant again. The mean rating was 4.16 (SD = 3.42). These central tendencies obscure the fact that 27% of the mothers believed that there was nothing at all they could do to improve their chances of a normal pregnancy or delivery in the future. The remaining mothers described a range of efficacious prevention options listed in Table 4.4.

To explore this further, we asked mothers who had perceived some control over their future childbearing to estimate the probability that they could prevent a recurrence of newborn intensive care if they did the things they mentioned and the probability of prevention if they did none of these things. As expected, the first probability (mean = 68.45%, SD = 26.06)

TABLE 4.4. Percentages of mothers reporting future efficacious preventions.

Activity	Percent
Any prevention effort	61.2
Engage in positive health behavior	34.3
Secure care for high-risk pregnancy	26.9
Avoid harmful substances	14.9
Reduce emotional stress	14.9
Quit work outside the home	11.9
Pay more attention to warning signals	11.9
Comply with medical advice	6.0
Curtail sexual intercourse	3.0

was significantly higher than the second probability (mean = 37.90, SD = 32.40). Twenty five percent of these mothers were certain that their failure to engage in these activities would guarantee a recurrence, and 17% were certain that they could avoid a recurrence by engaging in these activities.

Pregnancy Control Expectancies and Childbearing Plans

Trause and Kramer (1983) showed that mothers of premature infants, despite their higher risk for complicated pregnancies and deliveries, more rapidly attempted another pregnancy than did mothers of infants who were born healthy. They interpreted this finding as evidence of these mothers' overriding motivation to have a healthy pregnancy and delivery. They did not study, however, the psychological factors that might shape these mothers' childbearing decisions.

Six months after NICU discharge, mothers who were not currently pregnant (all but three) were asked to estimate the probability that they would try to have another child. The mean probability was 43.97% (SD = 42.10). Twenty-six percent of the mothers were convinced that they would try to have another child, contrasted to 34% percent who were sure that they would not try again. Seventy-eight percent of the mothers said that their decision to have another child was shaped to some extent by events that had already occurred. For example, 40% of the mothers said that they feared a recurrence of complications in future pregnancies and deliveries and they would not want to endure this experience again. For 20% of the mothers, recurrence was not a concern because they had already decided to limit their family to the current number of children. Half of the mothers said that their decision to have another child would be influenced by future events and circumstances. Thirteen percent stated that they would wait to see if their fears of a recurrence of pregnancy and delivery complications could be allayed by developments in obstetric care that could reduce their risk. Twenty-five percent said that practical and financial considerations in the future (e.g., money, housing, marital status) would influence their decision. Finally, 20% said they would defer any decision until their baby's development and health outcomes were known. Approximately 10% of the couples were so certain of their decision to forego future pregnancies that the wife was sterilized or the husband obtained a vasectomy.

Do mothers' appraisals of control and anticipated prevention activities figure in their childbearing plans? Before answering this question, we determined the effect of mothers' age, education, parity, and infants' medical severity on these variables. Mothers of first-born children were more certain that they would try to have another child and described more activities in their prevention plan. The same was true for the younger mothers, but the relation between parity and these expectations was independent of mothers' age. Mothers of sicker infants also described more prevention activities should they become pregnant again. The perceived control rating itself, however, was unrelated to background variables.

Without controlling for background variables, mothers who described more prevention activities did think that it was more likely that they would try to have another child. But, when statistical controls were instituted for these background variables, the relation bewteen prevention plans and the estimated likelihood of future pregnancies disappeared.

The same procedures were followed in examining the role of future pregnancy control and prevention activities in couples' permanent decision to forego future pregnancies through sterilization or vasectomy. Echoing the findings reported above, mothers of first-born children and younger mothers were less likely to adopt these permanent birth control procedures. In this case, the significant inverse relation between the rating of personal control over future pregnancy outcomes and the use of permanent birth control remained significant independent of the background variables. Thus, whereas the role of mothers' control and prevention appraisals in their intentions to attempt another pregnancy appear to be outweighed by their interest in having a larger family—as is implied by the effect of parity on their childbearing plans—the anticipation of the lack of control may have an impact on the decision of a relatively few couples to use permanent birth control to rule out a recurrence of problem pregnancies and deliveries.

Comforting Alternatives to the Perception of Personal Control

Burger (1989) notes a paradox in the literature on perceived control. On the one hand, the research documenting the benefits of perceiving control suggests that people will retain control rather than abandon their efforts to influence events whenever possible. But he also reviewed studies showing that people sometimes prefer to abandon control or react negatively to the circumstances in which they are expected to control the situation. Miller

(1979; 1980) proposed that people will prefer control over an aversive situation when they believe that harm is less likely by retaining than by giving up control. Miller hypothesized that surrendering control is especially likely in health-care situations because of the assumption that care providers are better able to effect control over the problem.

Mothers clearly differed in their *need* to assert control in one area—their child's medical care in the hospital. Asked to describe how much control they had wanted over their child's medical care and treatment and any consequences of their failure to gain needed control, 25% of the mothers mentioned their active participation in at least some decisions, as in "making suggestions that were carried out," "having my views on the course of treatment respected," and "feeling part of a partnership on behalf of my child." These mothers were not seeking primary control over the treatment itself. Rather, they were pursuing what Reid (1984) terms "participatory control" in the health-care process. This type of control emphasizes a cooperative partnership, in which the recipient concedes the competence of the care provider. The provider in turn provides information necessary for the recipient to make informed decisions about care and actively solicits the recipient's involvement in those decisions. The importance of participatory control has been demonstrated in studies of cancer patients (Weissman & Worden, 1976) and patients with heart disease (Boyd, Yeager, & McMillan, 1973). Participatory control has been shown to make a greater difference than personal control in adjusting to some health problems. particularly those that are chronic (Affleck et al., 1987; Reid, 1984). As might be expected, the mothers classified in this group were rarely critical of the NICU physicians' or nurses' willingness to share control over medical decision-making.

A second group of mothers, comprising roughly half the sample, appeared uninterested in acquiring a sense of participatory control. Instead, they remarked how they had willingly surrendered control over their child's treatment. Many in this category stressed the confidence they had in the staff's competence to make the best decisions on behalf of their child:

> I just didn't know what to do. But my baby had a very good doctor and I was reassured about the hospital, that it was the best place, and that if anything could be done, this was the place it would happen. Looking back, it was a good experience because the doctors and nurses were so good at their jobs.

> Whatever the doctors said to do, I tried to do. When they said not to worry, I didn't. And that worked out pretty well.

> Things really didn't bother me, because I knew he was in the best place in the state. I just kept reminding myself that the doctors would be able to take care of it all, and they did.

> After seeing what went on in the unit—the monitors, the respirators, the tube feedings—I became convinced that they could do what needed to be done, so I stopped feeling anxious.

> I never really worried, because all of the staff seemed so competent and experienced. I never felt that they couldn't handle any problem that came up.

> What I liked actually was that the doctors never told me what they were going to do. In case it didn't work, I didn't have to have my expectations shattered.

> The unit was phenomenal. I knew that I couldn't do what they could. I had all the confidence in the world in them, and that feeling helped me a lot.

These parents were comforted by a perception of "vicarious" control over their child's care and treatment (Rothbaum et al., 1982). Unlike the person who has gained a sense of participatory control, which emphasizes a cooperative partnership, the individual who pursues a sense of vicarious control relinquishes all control to the health-care provider.

A third group of mothers, comprising about 20% of the smaple, were unwilling to accord total control over their child's care to the NICU staff but had been unable to achieve a satisfying level of participatory control. These mothers were highly critical of the staff's perceived unwillingness to involve them in critical decisions, or even to inform them about treatment decisions that had already been made and carried out. The attitudes of the mothers quoted next exemplified this criticism:

> It was difficult for me to get the level of communication with the doctors that I wanted without sensing a lot of resentment from them. I can understand why doctors say "Just trust me, I'm the professional and I'll take care of you"; they are trying to reassure you. But the people I've known who have serious medical problems and have done the best are the ones who are the most aggressive with the doctors. They get the information they need, they challenged the doctor on every detail, and they really participated in their own care. I think the doctor's role should be to give information and to help you make the decision rather than to make the decision for you. Sometimes I got the impression that the doctors were trying to put something over on me. While the quality of care was excellent, the bad thing was how hard you had to fight to get the information. In the end, I think my persistence really improved the quality of my baby's care.

> We never had much of a say in what was done. I never remember being asked "should we do this?" I would like to have at least been told about things before they happened rather than after the fact. We got a bill for her eye exam and we weren't even told the results! We always got answers when we called on the phone, but just once I wish someone had called us to give us information before we asked.

> Just before I took her home, I found out that she had an episode of hemorrhaging in the brain. The doctor never said anything about it at the time. Now I wonder if there's anything else wrong that someone forgot to tell me.

> The unit was very confusing, total chaos, with people running around and monitors going off all over the place. Our goal was to learn as much as we could about what was going on. I wanted information on my child's blood type but they said they were so busy they couldn't get me the information. Although they never said it, I think most of the doctors would like to kick the parents out of the unit.

These individual differences in parents' need for personal control over their child's medical care, the comforting alternatives of participatory and vicarious control, and the consequences of these appraisals for parent–professional relationships in the hospital merit special scrutiny in our efforts to understand the alternative pathways to coping with this and other medical crises. Not all parents wanted to participate in medical decisions involving their child. But, for those who did, the response of health-care providers was a critical factor in their appraisals of the parent–professional relationship. As we will demonstrate further in chapter 8, where we review mothers' remembrances of the hospitalization, these appraisals remain a key feature of mothers' longer term response to newborn intensive care.

Positive Outcome Expectancies

As noted previously, mothers who had been unable to imagine ways in which they could control the outcomes of future pregnancies may have been comforted by expecting positive outcomes nonetheless. There is mounting evidence, however, that what people expect from the future does not necessarily depend on their perceived ability to control events (see Scheier & Carver, 1987 for a review). That is, some individuals expect good things to happen, whether or not they believe they can make them happen. Unwarranted optimism may be an illusion every bit as adaptive as the illusion of control (Taylor & Brown, 1988).

At NICU discharge, mothers estimated the chances, from 0% to 100%, that their child's future health and development "would be normal in all respects." The average mother estimated a 75% probability of a normal outcome, but there was substantial variability in their estimates (SD = 25.06%). Approximately 24% of the mothers had no doubt that their child would be normal; only 7% thought that there was greater than a 50/50 chance of problems. Problems that mothers were even slightly concerned might develop are listed in Table 4.5. Clearly, the lagest proportion of mothers were concerned about the possibility of a significant delay in their child's development that might be a sign of mental retardation.

Neither a mother's age, education, or parity, nor the severity of her infant's medical problems figured in her estimate of the probability of a

TABLE 4.5. Concerns expressed by mothers about their infant's future health and development.

Concern	Percent
Any concerns	75.9
Developmental delay or mental retardation	43.8
Motor disability	23.2
Sensory disability	19.6
Chronic or acute medical problems	17.0
Growth problem	6.3
Behavioral or emotional problems	1.8

normal outcome. Mothers' outcome expectancies were unrelated to their control perceptions at either hospital discharge or 6 months later. At the same time, those who expected a better outcome reported more positive mood at hospital discharge ($r = .21, p < .05$) 6 months after discharge ($r = .24, p < .05$), and 18 months after discharge ($r = .30, p < .05$). Because of the high correlations among mood reports over time, the predictive relation between mothers' mood and global distess was not significant when earlier mood was partialled from the associations. It is possible, therefore, that the comforting effects of mothers' expectations of a good outcome remain with them for many months after discharge.

An especially intriguing finding was that mothers who were more confident about their child's normal development had children who in fact exhibited more favorable cognitive and adaptive behavior outcomes 18 months later ($r = .36, p < .001$). Even controlling for background variables, mothers' mood at discharge, and mothers' perceptions of control in the hospital, this remained a significant association.

We were unable to uncover any evidence for confounding or intervening variables that might account for this predictive association. Within the limits of the variables measured, this relation was not due to the possibilities that these mothers had infants who had less severe early medical problems, enjoyed greater emotional well-being, viewed themselves as better caregivers, felt closer to their child, exhibited more responsiveness with their child, or perceived greater control over their child's outcomes. In the previous chapter on the search for meaning, we reported that mothers who had perceived no benefits in the crisis also had children who showed less positive developmental outcomes. These mothers also felt less optimistic about the chances that their child's outcome would be normal. Thus, mothers may find it easier to find benefits when they believe more strongly that the future holds good things for their child. Yet, even when the perception of benefits was taken into account, the relation between positive outcome expectancies and actual outcomes was still significant.

Outcome Expectancies and Dispositional Optimism

Recent research on dispositional optimism offers one interpretation of our findings on the benefits of mothers' positive outcome expectancies. Scheier and Carver (1987) theorize that people who are dispositionally optimistic, that is, people who have a generalized expectancy for positive outcomes, are protected against the negative consequences of stressful experiences. They reviewed evidence that dispositionally optimistic individuals are better able to adjust to threatening experiences, are physically healthier, and recover more quickly from medical procedures. In addition, these benefits of optimism do not rely on the perception of personal control over the outcomes of these stressors.

Could mothers who are dispositionally optimistic be the ones who expected a better outcome for their child? We cannot say without a separate measure of this propensity. But, it is clear that these mothers' expectancies were not shaped by a host of objective indicators of their child's risk for future problems. This at least allows room for personal dispositions to influence their expectations. According to Scheier and Carver (1987), one reason why optimists appear better adapted to threatening experiences is that their expectation of a positive outcome encourages them to take direct actions to improve their situation. Yet, our measure of mothers' tendency to engage in problem-solving activities as a way of coping with their child's hospitalization (which we describe in Chapter 6) did not relate to mothers' optimism about their child's future. It is still possible, of course, that these mothers were better able to solve any child-care problems they encountered later. One can imagine a scenario in which optimistic mothers might be less apt to be demoralized by these difficulties. If they continue to perceive their child as "normal" and continue to expect a positive outcome despite emergent problems, they may find it easier to take actions that could actually improve the outcome.

This line of reasoning is consistent with research on the "fragile child syndrome," a term that characterizes parents' perceptions of previously ill, but now healthy, children as frail and in need of protection (Green & Solint, 1964). Compared to mothers of healthy-born infants, mothers of premature infants, especially those with perinatal medical problems, tend to see their child as weaker and in greater danger of dying (DiVitto & Goldberg, 1979; Plunkett et al., 1986) and are more concerned about such matters as their child's appetite, risk of injury, and physical strength (Perrin et al., 1989). Mothers who view their prematurely born youngsters as being more vulnerable for health problems may well encounter difficulty in setting age-appropriate limits, accounting for the established link between vulnerable child perceptions and behavioral problems surrounding peer relationships and self-control among preschoolers who were prematurely born (Perrin et al., 1989).

Our findings on mothers' search for mastery over the crisis of newborn intensive care are complex and capture the many nuances in the literature on the advantages and disadvantages of perceived control. Several key distinctions are warranted by our analysis: (a) differences in perceived control over different outcomes; (b) differences among retrospective control appraisals, control expectancies, and outcome expectancies; and (c) variations in the need for control over children's medical care in the hospital. In the next chapter, we continue our analysis of the search for meaning and mastery by considering the implications of mothers' search for a cause of their infant's premature delivery and medical problems. As we demonstrate, some mothers were able to restore a belief in a controllable future by explaining the past.

5
The Search for Causes

In the preceding two chapters, we discussed how parents are able to restore a sense of meaning and mastery in the unfolding crisis of newborn intensive care. Next, we explore how the search for meaning and mastery can be aided by parents' ability to find a cause of their infant's medical problems. It is crucial to recognize that the causes of a premature or hazardous delivery are, in individual cases, difficult to identify with much certainty. Thus, physicians and other health professionals may be unable or unwilling to provide a confident answer to parents who are searching for a specific cause. Nonetheless, as we demonstrate in this chaper, most parents construct their own causal theories. We discuss how some of their theories seem to aid their adaptation whereas others seem to impede it.

Causal Searching

From the very beginning, I was trying to find out why this happened. The fact that I couldn't find any answers made this whole situation even more difficult. If we had an answer, our baby's hospitalization would have been easier to cope with.

As this parent admits, the failure to find a cause of this event can make it more aversive. How much were mothers thinking about the causes of their infant's medical problems during the hospital stay? At hospital discharge, they reported on four-point scales how much they were currently searching for causes and how much they had been soon after their infant's admission to the NICU. Mothers said they had been thinking more about the causes soon after the admission than currently. Whereas one third of the mothers said that they had been searching for causes almost constantly in the time after admission, fewer than 10% were doing so at the time of discharge. Conversely, at discharge, 30% said that they were not thinking about causes, compared with only 13% who reported not thinking about causes during the time just after the admission. As we document next, most mothers were able to identify one or more causes of this event before taking their baby home from the hospital.

A Taxonomy of Causal Beliefs

We used several approaches to assess mothers' beliefs about the causes of their infant's premature delivery, subsequent medical problems, or both. The first was the inspection of "spontaneous" causal ascriptions that mothers made at the beginning of the interview, when they were asked simply to "describe the crisis of newborn intensive care." We thought it critical to establish that our subsequent direct inquiry into mothers' causal beliefs would be eliciting more than a quick judgment of the plausibility of the causal factors. If causal perceptions emerged in these descriptions, we would have stronger confirmation of their salience in mothers' response to this event. In fact, 61% of the mothers did make an unprompted statement about the causes of their child's problems. Most of these parents cited a physical cause, for example, toxemia or cervical incompetence. One in five mothers also expressed a suspicion that it was something they did or did not do that caused this to happen. A smaller number raised the possibility that their obstetrician was at fault in some way.

We also asked mothers directly what, if anything, health professionals had told them about causes. Next, we asked them to summarize any other causal factors they thought might have been at least in part responsible for these events. In an earlier study (Affleck et al., 1982a), we showed that many mothers often mentioned behavioral (distal) causes only after they were asked to account for factors that may have been responsible for biomedical (proximal) causes of a premature delivery. Because such distal causes seem to carry greater weight in the search for mastery and meaning, we asked mothers whether any causal factors mentioned might themselves have a cause. Finally, they rated the importance of each 12 categories of possible causal factors that we derived from our earlier research. The categories presented to mothers are identified below, along with examples of specific causes that mothers assigned to each category when they made their ratings.

1. *Something the mother did or did not do* (e.g., poor diet, failing to take prescribed vitamins, not enough sleep, too much housework, smoking, drinking alcohol, bowling the night before the delivery, too much aerobics, did not insist on inducing labor, did not pick the right obstetrician)
2. *Something someone else did or did not do* (e.g., obstetrician was not available at the time of the delivery, husband too demanding, doctor did not treat toxemia aggressively enough)
3. *A chronic illness or disorder predating the pregnancy* (e.g., high blood pressure, anemia, chronic infections)
4. *An acute illness or infection during the pregnancy* (e.g., caught the flu, had a urinary tract infection)
5. *The mother's age* (i.e., too young or too old)

6. *The mother's personality characteristics* (e.g., too hard driving, a constant worrier)
7. *Factors in the physical environment* (e.g., lives near a toxic waste site, chemicals used at work, exposure to x rays at work)
8. *Stressful situations* (e.g., death of grandmother, husband losing job, moving to new house, difficulties with in-laws)
9. *Surgery or medical procedures before the delivery* (e.g., cervical repair, appendectomy, gall bladder removal)
10. *Medical complications of the pregnancy* (e.g., toxemia, incompetent cervix, placental dysfunction)
11. *Genetic factors/family history* (e.g., premature births run in the family)
12. *Chance* (e.g., just a one in million chance)

The complexity of many mothers' causal explanation is conveyed in the following excerpts:

To begin with, I had an incompetent cervix. . . But there were a lot of things I shouldn't have done, like working in the yard too much, not quitting smoking. . . Also, the night before the delivery, I had intercourse. . . I also had pneumonia four years ago and that might have weakened me. . . There's probably something about my personality that prevented me from following the advice I was getting on taking it easier. . . Sometimes I wonder about whether our well water is contaminated. . . There's a lot of emotional stress at work and that might have been a factor. . . I did have an incompetent cervix, or so I was told.

I don't think my diet was good enough, and perhaps I overdid it by traveling too much on my vacation. . . I'm the type who tries to handle too many things on my own, and maybe that prevented me from taking things easier. . . I also think that my obstetrician didn't treat my toxemia aggressively enough. . . I was exposed to potentially harmful chemicals at work. . . During my pregnancy I was under a lot of stress after my grandmother died and because of problems I was having with my inlaws. . . Also, two my sisters also had premature deliveries.

I think I worked too hard and too long. . . I should have quit work before this happened. . . Also, I have a very nervous personality and that makes it hard for me to relax. . . My life was very stressful during the pregnancy—a lot of problems at work, my husband's career change, the fact that I wasn't thrilled with being pregnant. . . Maybe my allergies played a part, and there is a history of eclampsia in the family.

Even though I cut back, I still smoked some during the pregnancy and did drink some beer and wine from time to time. . . The night before the delivery I went bowling, and that might have damaged something. . . My husband wasn't supportive or dependable enough. . . I have a thyroid condition and caught a virus. . . I wonder about whether my two miscarriages might have created a physical problem.

We were impressed too with the extent to which several fathers went to explain the causes of this event:

My wife smoked during the pregnancy. . . She didn't take the vitamins she was advised to take. . . She's too sensitive, too much a worrier. . . She had a lot of emotional stress at work. . . We had sex the night before the delivery. . . She had some bleeding during the first trimester, and I don't think the doctor checked her enough after this happened. . . I also wonder about the quality of the water we're drinking. . . She did have an infection during the pregnancy, too.

My wife continued working, but I was also responsible because I didn't discourage this. . . She took a lot of medications just before she became pregnant. . . She had a flu during her pregnancy. . . I have a very uptight personality and that makes my wife nervous. . . I also wonder about additives in the food. . . She had some medical tests during the pregnancy for a gastrointestinal problem. . . It might be that the baby was very active before the delivery and might have torn the membranes.

I think I placed too much stress on my wife. . . I didn't help around the house as much as I should. . . Maybe the pressure I was under at work made me too short-tempered with her. . . The obstetrician didn't follow my wife's condition closely enough. . . There was a gas leak in the house. . . My mother-in-law took DES and that might have created problems with my wife's cervix.

In our statistical analyses, we preserved the distinctions mothers had made among certain types of behavioral causes and the identities of other individuals whose behavior was judged to be causal. Table 5.1 presents the proportion of mothers who rated each of the resulting 20 factors as being

TABLE 5.1. Distribution of mothers' causal explanations.

Category	Not a cause (%)	Minor cause (%)	Major cause (%)
Biomedical factors	24.6	14.0	61.4
Pregnancy complications	41.2	6.1	52.6
Chronic health problem	79.8	12.3	7.9
Acute illness/infection	81.6	9.6	8.8
Prior surgery	91.2	1.8	7.0
Own behavior	33.3	23.7	43.9
Harmful habits	76.3	8.8	14.9
Poor health behavior	73.7	8.8	17.5
Hazardous activity	84.2	8.8	7.0
Physical strain	64.0	15.8	20.2
Poor health care monitoring	93.9	1.8	4.4
Other behavior	90.4	3.5	6.1
Other person's behavior	67.5	9.6	22.8
Obstetrician	80.7	7.0	12.3
Child's father	91.2	3.5	5.3
Other health professional	93.0	3.5	3.5
Other person	93.9	1.8	4.4
Psychological stress	51.8	14.9	33.3
Chance	43.9	33.3	22.8
Own personality traits	72.8	10.5	16.7
Familial/hereditary factors	73.7	13.2	13.2
Physical environment	84.2	12.3	3.5
Age	89.5	7.9	2.6

"not a cause," "a minor cause," or "a major cause." Not surprisingly, three fourths of the mothers thought that biomedical factors played a causal role in the outcome, and more than half viewed complications of pregnancy as a causal factor. More surprising perhaps was that two thirds of the mothers attributed this outcome or the biomedical cause to their own behavior, mentioning harmful habits, poor health behavior, engaging in a discrete hazardous activity, physical strain, failing to monitor their health care adequately, and other unclassifiable behaviors.

Many mothers volunteered how they maintained these "self-attributions" despite their own and others' efforts to minimize them. The mothers quoted below described this process and the reasons underlying their reluctance to abandon this causal ascription. Their comments reveal how attributions to their own behavior can support efforts to regain control:

> In the beginning, people warned me not to go over and over in my mind what I might have done to bring about the premature labor. At first, I told myself that I wouldn't let myself think that. I would tell myself that I had a healthy pregnancy, I took good care of myself, etc. I wanted to believe that this was just an unfortunate accident. But as time went on, I couldn't stop thinking about what I might have done to cause this. *I guess I needed to know that there was a cause and that maybe next time it could be different.*

> I do blame myself for what happened even though the doctors and nurses kept telling me I had nothing to do with it. *If I could find something that I did to cause*

TABLE 5.2. Percentages of mothers reporting that health professionals were the source of their causal explanations.

Category	Percent of total	Percent of those citing this cause
Biomedical factors		
Pregnancy complications	52.1	87.4
Chronic health problem	4.3	21.3
Acute illness/infection	2.1	10.4
Prior surgery	2.1	21.9
Own behavior		
Harmful habits	0.0	0.0
Poor health behavior	4.3	11.5
Hazardous activity	4.3	23.8
Physical strain	2.1	6.0
Poor health care monitoring	0.0	0.0
Other person's behavior		
Obstetrician	1.1	5.4
Child's father	0.0	0.0
Other health professional	1.1	20.8
Psychological stress	0.0	0.0
Chance/bad luck	9.7	29.3
Own personality traits	0.0	0.0
Familial/hereditary factors	1.1	19.1
Physical environment	1.1	7.4
Age	0.0	0.0

this, I think I'd feel better, because then I'd know what to do to prevent it from happening again if I decide to have other children.

One third of the mothers described another person's behavior as a causal factor, most frequently citing errors in their obstetrician's judgment or practice. Another common attribution was to stressful events, identified as a cause by half the mothers. Slightly fewer than 60% of the mothers attributed the event to chance.

Each of these causal factors was also analyzed in relation to what mothers said they had been told by health professionals about the causes of the event (see Table 5.2). There were only two causal factors that more than 5% of the mothers reported had been communicated to them by health-care providers. Fifty-two percent stated that they had been told that the premature delivery or the infant's medical problem was caused by medical complications of the pregnancy, and 10% stated that they had been told that the problem was owing to chance. Apparently, the other frequent attributions such as those to one's own behavior or to stressful events were typically not the result of mothers' communications with physicians or nurses.

In the remainder of this chapter, we summarize additional findings on two relatively common causal ascriptions: (a) mothers attributions to their own behavior, and (b) mothers' attributions to other people's behavior. We discuss how certain self-attributions can assist mothers' adaption and how attributions to other people can threaten it. Before summarizing our findings on self-attributions, we provide some background on the psychological meaning of this type of causal explanation.

Two Types of Self-Blame for Aversive Events

In 1977, Bulman and Wortman published a pivotal investigation of people's attributions of blame and their adjustment to serious accidents that left them paralyzed. A key finding of their study is that victims who believed that they acted in some way to cause their accident appeared to their care providers to be coping more successfully with their paralysis. Later, Janoff-Bulman (1979) delineated more fully the reasons why certain types of self-blame may assist people's adaptation to negative life events. She distinguished two forms of self-blame. The first she called *behavioral self-blame* because it involves the attribution of undesirable events to one's own modifiable behavior. This type of self-blame may increase one's faith that future negative events remain under personal control and can help to restore assumptions threatened by the event:

> By blaming oneself behaviorally—that is, because of something one specifically did or failed to do...the victim is able to retain prior beliefs. The victim can continue to believe in a world in which outcomes are controllable and therefore meaningful ("I am good; I simply did a foolish thing"), and in which the world

can still be perceived as benevolent, for the victim can minimize the likelihood of future occurrences of such negative outcomes" (Janoff-Bulman, 1989, p. 165).

Janoff-Bulman termed the second form of self-blame *characterological self-blame*, because it involves attributions to stable aspects of the self. With this type of self-blame, negative events are seen as the result of personal deficiencies that are presumably more immutable, and the prospects of influencing the future are less favorable.

Bulman and Wortman's provocative and perhaps counterintuitive finding spawned a series of studies that examined the role of self-blame in adapting to threatening events. Characterological self-blame has been linked with poorer adaptation to abortion (Mueller & Major, 1989), rape (Meyer & Taylor, 1986), and breast cancer (Timko & Janoff-Bulman, 1985). The statistical relation between self-blame and adaptation, however, has been inconsistent across these studies. Behavioral self-blame has been associated with positive adaptation among rape victims (Janoff-Bulman, 1979), children and adolescents with diabetes (Tennen, Affleck, Allen, McGrade, & Ratzan, 1984), individuals with smell disorders (Tennen et al., in press), and women with breast cancer (Timko & Janoff-Bulman, 1985). Behavioral self-blame was shown to be unrelated to adaptation in studies of patients with kidney disease (Witenberg, Blanchard, Suls, Tennen, McCoy, & McGoldrick, 1983), another group of women with breast cancer (Taylor et al., 1984), and mothers of diabetic children (Affleck et al., 1985). And, in one study of rape victims (Meyer & Taylor, 1986) and in two studies of accident victims (Frey, Rogner, Schuler, & Korte, 1985; Nielson & McDonald, 1988), it was related to poorer adaptation.

Consequences of Self-Attributions

In an earlier study of mothers whose infants had been treated on the same newborn intensive care unit from which our current sample was drawn (Tennen et al., 1986), we examined relations among the severity of the child's medical problems, mothers' behavioral self-blame for the problem, mothers' perception of personal control (over the infant's recovery and future development, and the recurrence of the problem in future pregnancies), and mothers' mood in the first 3 months after hospital discharge. Several predictions flowing from Janoff-Bulman's theory of self-blame and Walster's (1966) and Shaver's (1970) works on defensive attribution were tested.

First, we hypothesized that mothers whose children were more ill, as we had found in a study of mothers of children with diabetes (Affleck et al.,

1985), would be likely to engage in behavioral self-blame in order to reassure themselves that outcomes were still a function of their own behavior. This prediction was confirmed by a significant relation between mother's perceived severity of the problem and the extent to which she ascribed the cause of the problem to her own behavior. Findings from the current sample show that our objective measure of the severity of the child's medical problems also correlates with the extent to which mothers attributed the problem to their own behavior.

We also predicted that behavioral self-blame would be linked to perceptions of greater personal control over the important outcomes of this event. This hypothesis was supported by significant relations between the magnitude of mother's behavioral self-blame and their perceptions of personal control over their child's recovery and their future childbearing outcomes. In turn, mothers' perceptions of control over recurrence were associated with more positive mood states. A path analysis was conducted to see whether the data were consistent with the following model: mothers of sicker infants would be more likely to blame themselves in order to increase their confidence that they could prevent a recurrence in future pregnancies, which would, in turn, predict more positive mood. The findings of the path analysis confirmed the tenability of this model as one explanation of the data.

To explore further the relation between attributions and control in the current sample, we inspected the correlations between various attributions and mothers' ratings of their ability to prevent a recurrence of problems with future pregnancies and deliveries and the number of activities they mentioned in their prevention plan (see Chapter 4). These findings, presented in Table 5.3, show that mothers who attributed the problem to harmful habits, inadequate health behaviors, physical strain, and stress

TABLE 5.3. Correlations of selected causal attributions with mothers' perceived control over future pregnancies, number of future prevention activities, and the perceived avoidability of their infant's medical problems.

Attribution	Perceived control	Prevention activities	Avoidability of problem
Harmful habits	.30**	.40**	.05
Poor health behavior	.38**	.42**	.12
Hazardous activity	.06	.14	.14
Poor health care monitoring	.20*	.05	.16
Physical strain	.31**	.43**	.14
Psychological stress	.28**	.41**	.17
Own personality	.12	.09	.12
Obstetric error	.13	.11	.25*
Chance	−.30**	−.23*	−.21*

* $p < .05$.
** $p < .01$.

perceived more control over, and thought they could do more to prevent problems with, future pregnancies. Recall that in Chapter 4, we reported that efforts to modify these causal factors were, in fact, mentioned by mothers as ways of avoiding a recurrence.

Consistent with theory (Janoff-Bulman, 1979), attributions to stable personality characteristics were unrelated to control and prevention appraisals. As expected, mothers who thought that the problem was caused more by chance perceived less control over the outcomes of future pregnancies and enumerated fewer ways in which they could avoid a recurrence. Blaming the obstetrician for the outcome did not correlate with these control appraisals.

Table 5.3 also presents the relations between causal attributions and mothers retrospective appraisals of the avoidability of the problem. The latter variable was measured by the question: "Knowing what you know today, to what extent do you believe that your baby's medical problems could have been avoided?" Responses were made on a scale ranging from 0 = at all avoidable to 10 = completely avoidable. One interesting finding is that mothers who engaged in behavioral self-blame for the outcome were not more likely to view the problem as having been avoidable. On the other hand, mothers who attributed the outcome to obstetric errors did regard it as having been more avoidable. The significance of these two findings are discussed more completely in the following sections.

Behavioral Self-Blame and Guilt

Although behavioral selff-blame may be adaptive to the extent that it buttresses the belief in a controllable future, some writers have interpreted this attribution as a sign of damaging guilt in parents of sick or developmentally disabled children (e.g., Mintzer, Als, Tronick, & Brazelton, 1985; Trout, 1983). Accordingly, we decided to explore some of the potential maladaptive consequences of this attribution. At NICU discharge, we asked mothers if they had felt guilty over feelings of responsibility for their infant's problems. Approximately two thirds of the mothers answered that they had. And those who had ascribed a greater causal role to their own behavior were in fact more likely to report guilty feelings.

Yet, by discharge, most mothers reported a decline in feelings of guilt, and at least by hospital discharge, these mothers' mood reports did not differ significantly from mothers who had reported no guilt since the delivery. We suspect that most of these "guilty" mothers were able to avoid psychological harm because they were able to cope effectively with this emotion. In fact, 90% of them described at least one factor that helped them mitigate their guilt. The most common one, reported by 56% of the guilty mothers, was obtaining "absolution" from friends and family, as in "being told that it wasn't my fault." Thirty-two percent said they benefited from reminding themselves that they were not at fault. Fifteen percent focused on their child's progress as a way of minimizing their guilt. Twelve percent stated that they dealt with their guilt by expressing their emotions about it, and the same proportion said they were helped by making reparations, such as "concentrating all my attention on the baby," and "going to visit every day." Finally, 8% described efforts to avoid thinking about their role in the problem as a way of dealing with their guilt. To illustrate, the mothers quoted next were able to contend with their disturbing feelings of responsibility for the problem by concentrating on their responsibility for the solution:

> Even though my doctors and nurses kept telling me I had nothing to do with it, I blame myself. Since I was the one who put her there, I can't walk away from it. I'm doing the best I can to help her through this and to see that nothing else goes wrong.

> At times I wanted to run away from it all. . . I was feeling so bad that I might have put her in this awful situation. But it's also my responsibility to see that she gets through this and that nothing more happens to her. For my own sanity, I need to know that I was always there for her in the hospital, that I did everything I could to help.

We suspected further that when mothers knew they might be posing a risk to the pregnancy by engaging in a behavior and when that behavior could have been avoided, they might suffer most from their sense of responsibility for this outcome. Therefore, we questioned mothers who had ascribed their infant's problems to their own behavior about these appraisals. Collapsing across all self-behavior attributions, most mothers in this group did report a moderate level of prior concern about the consequences of their behavior for the pregnancy. The two behaviors that had elicited the greatest concern were engaging in harmful habits such as smoking and drinking and failing to engage in healthful behaviors such as exercising and following a nutritious diet.

But the potential emotional distress associated with these mothers' forewarning may have been alleviated by the perceived difficulty of making behavorial changes. No mother reported that a change in the behavior in question would have been easy. In fact, almost half said that it would have been extremely difficult, if not impossible, to make such a change. They viewed their capacity to make changes in their level of physical activity at home or at work as having been most limited. Most of the mothers who ascribed the outcome to excessive physical strain pointed to the impossibility of making other arrangements to perform household chores or physically demanding child-rearing activities or to change the conditions of the workplace. These findings help to explain why, as stated previously, self attributions did not correlate with the perceived avoidability of the problem.

The Emotional Costs of Blaming Others

So far, we have underscored the adaptive value of parents' ability to identify a cause of their infant's need to be hospitalized on the newborn intensive care unit. To conclude, however, that *any* causal attribution is helpful would be inaccurate. In this section we describe the emotional costs of one causal belief expressed by a sizeable minority of parents—the perception that other people, usually the mother's obstetrician, were responsible for this outcome.

Among the attributions we have discussed, one unique consequence of holding the obstetrician responsible for this event was stated previously: the perception that the problem could have been avoided. In our inquiry into causal beliefs, we had also asked parents about the causal sufficiency of factors they thought to be responsible for the problem. Put briefly, was the factor mentioned sufficient alone to have caused this outcome? Nearly 90% of the mothers who blamed their obstetrician thought that it was. To no other factor did more than half of the mothers accord such causal sufficiency. Thus, mothers who blamed their obstetrician were not only more inclined to view their baby's need for intensive care as being avoidable but believed that if the doctor had acted otherwise it could have been prevented.

In our previous longitudinal studies of mothers of intensive-care–treated infants, we discovered consistently negative consequences of blaming others for this event (Affleck et al., 1982a; Affleck et al., 1985; Tennen et al., 1986). These consequences included greater mood disturbance and expected caretaking problems at hospital discharge, greater reported care-taking problems 9 months after discharge, and less optimal interactions with the child 18 months after discharge. In the current study, mothers who blamed others reported more psychological distress 18 months after discharge ($r = .24$, $p < .05$), and did so regardless of background variables and mothers' mood measured at NICU discharge.

We have reviewed the literature on causal attributions for misfortune and located 25 studies that examined the relation between blaming others and adaptation (Tennen & Affleck, in press). A wide spectrum of stressful events were examined in these studies. They include, among others, victims of fires, accidents, and natural disasters, patients with acute or chronic illnesses, women who had had an abortion or suffered a miscarriage, and individuals who were grieving the loss of a parent. In 80% of these studies, blaming someone else for the problem was related to poorer adaptation. Next, we review several possible explanations of this consistent finding, emphasizing their application to mothers of medically fragile infants.

The Psychodynamic Explanation

Whether informed by traditional psychoanalytic thinking (Fenichel, 1945; Freud, 1923; Meissner, 1978), object relations theory (Kernberg, 1975;

Klein, 1964), or self-psychology (Kohut, 1977), psychodynamic theorists share the view that some people bring to threatening life situations a developmental vulnerability that accounts for adaptational difficulties. What these perspectives share is the view that blaming others and poor coping are part of the same deficit in personality structure. The interested reader may wish to review Sullivan's (1956) description of the "paranoid dynamism," Phillips' (1968) discussion of "turning against others," and Vaillant's (1977) taxonomy of immature defenses against anxiety for insights into this explanation of the link between other-blame and adaptational deficits.

It is difficult to assess the utility of this perspective for the explanation of our findings and those of broader literature on blaming others for misfortune. In none of these studies were psychodynamic hypotheses tested directly. More important, in none were assessments of personality taken before the occurrence of the threatening event or the onset of the chronic stressor.

A key finding in the empirical literature does pose a serious challenge to this explanation. Why does the prevalence of blaming others differ so greatly across types of misfortune? In the current study, almost one third of the mothers blamed someone else for the outcome, but in our study of mothers of diabetic children (Affleck et al., 1985), no mother blamed someone else for her child's condition. Apparently, there are either important situational differences that make other-blame more or less likely or, if the psychodynamic explanation is accurate, mothers of medically fragile infants possessed more primitive personality structures than mothers of diabetic children. The difficulty in arguing the latter proposition raises questions about the developmental diathesis perspective on blaming others.

The Loss of Control

If, as we have previously discussed, self-blame can reinforce a sense of personal control over the consequences or recurrence of a threatening event, might blaming others undercut a sense of control? Unfortunately, the literature contains few analyses of the relations among blaming others, perceived control, and well-being. Timko and Janoff-Bulman (1985) found that for mastectomy patients, the relation between blaming others and impaired adaptation was mediated by the belief that the surgery was unsuccessful rather than the perception of control over future health. In our study of men who had a heart attack (Affleck, Tennen, Croog, & Levine, 1987b), we found that those who blamed others for the attack perceived less control over future attacks but had no evidence that control perceptions or blaming others influenced well-being. And, in both the current and previous studies of mothers of medically fragile infants (Tennen et al., 1986), blaming others was unrelated to perceptions of control. Thus, despite the intuitive appeal of this explanation, there is little evidence that can be garnered for its support.

Shattered Illusions

Janoff-Bulman and Frieze (1983) and Perloff (1983) offer another explanation by which blaming others may interfere with people's adaptation to stressful events. They argue that illusions of invulnerability are shattered by victimization, and that "human-induced" events are especially likely to threaten well-being because "the victim is no longer able to feel secure in the world of other people" (Janoff-Bulman & Frieze, 1983, p. 5). Being harmed by another person highlights the fact that some people cannot be trusted. This revelation might be especially devastating when the other person is a trusted physician. As one of the mothers in our study remarked:

> My obstetrician kept trying to convince me that this was just a freak thing. But she also said that if I were to become pregnant again she would schedule a C section 2 weeks before my due date. Now I'm beginning to think that she could have done something different to prevent what happened. Maybe because my baby is sick, I have to blame somebody. But, looking back, I never did trust that doctor.

Unfortunately, the evidence supporting this explanation is largely anecdotal. But the literature on crime victims (Bard & Sangry, 1979; Scheppele & Bart, 1983) suggests that blaming other people for one's misfortune does shatter illusions of invulnerability, which in turn leads to a sense of helplessness, overwhelming anxiety, and other manifestations of distress.

The Failure of Vicarious Control

Rothbaum et al. (1982) contend that when people believe that important outcomes in their lives are controlled by other people, they are not necessarily helpless and demoralized. Rather, they can derive comfort in the perception of "vicarious control." In Chapter 4, we illustrated how the perception of vicarious control figured in some parents' willingness to surrender decisions about their child's care to physicians and nurses working on the NICU. It may also be true that the failure of vicarious control over the outcomes of the pregnancy occasions both blaming others and maladaptation.

Vicarious control is viewed by Rothbaum et al. as a "secondary" control strategy, more likely to be followed when attempts at personal, or "primary," control have failed or would be fruitless. When a vicarious control strategy fails, a need for retribution or justice could stall further efforts at cognitive adaptation. This might be true, for example, when the physician is perceived as having been able, but unwilling, to act in a more helpful manner. One parent's comments, excerpted previously in Chapter 1, are repeated here to illustrate this point:

> What happened to my child simply should not have happened. If he was born deformed, that's one thing. But my son's problem is something that could have been prevented and should have been prevented. He missed something. He knew better. I don't think I'll ever get over this fact.

Even in the absense of malice, the failure of a powerful other to act in one's perceived best interests can be devastating because it forces a major change in the meaning people attribute to their misfortune. The failure of this fallback position, and the resulting inclination to blame the other, may so undercut one's view of oneself and the world that attempts to restore meaning may be unsuccessful. Indeed, mothers who blamed their obstetricians were more likely to state that nothing good had come from this experience and that there was no purpose or satisfying reason for their misfortune. Although it may be harder for some parents to find meaning because they blame others, the mother quoted next blamed her doctor because she had not found a satisfying reason for her child's premature delivery:

> Why did our baby have to be born premature and be so sick? I can't understand why this happened to us. It's natural to want to find reasons for things, and when you can't, you end up picking on somebody. So, I guess that's why I'm feeling that the doctor was at fault for what happened.

A logical question flowing from this explanation is what effect blaming the obstetrician for the problem might have on mothers' relationship with physicians working on the NICU. In Chapter 4, we noted that a substantial minority of mothers criticized the failure of neonatologists to keep them adequately informed about, or to involve them in, decisions made about their child's care. We did find that mothers who blamed the obstetrician for the outcome were more likely to describe these difficulties with their child's physicians. Thus, another reason why the failure of vicarious control might lead to blaming others and poor adaptation is that some mothers generalized their distrust to other physicians caring for their child. In so doing, they may have cut themselves off from a key source of support during their child's hospitalization.

In ending this section, we must raise the possibility that blaming others is simply more plausible in certain situations, or taken a step further, just reflects people's accurate appraisals of the causes of the situation. Perhaps people who correctly conclude that someone else was the cause of their adversity are angry with the other person, and measures of psychological distress simply tap this hostility. Further psychological explanations might be unnecessary. Do our findings merely reflect the fact that in certain instances the obstetrician was blameworthy? Despite the pragmatic appeal of this idea, our experience with victimized individuals suggests that there is more psychological meaning to other-blame beyond what is "real," and that people actively create the realities to which they then respond. We have been impressed with people's tendency to see others as the cause of their misfortune or to avoid this attribution despite objective circumstances. Consider, as a postscript to this section, that the mother quoted below, who readily could have blamed her obstetrician, blamed herself instead:

> When I began to notice that I was starting to go into labor, I called my doctor and he advised me to wait it out and to call him later. As things turned out, my water broke, and I had to take an ambulance to the hospital. But really, I think it was my fault. I should have insisted that he do something about it right away.

Health-care professionals, when telling mothers about the causes of their infants' medical problems, rarely mentioned more than complications of the pregnancy or their random occurence. With this limited information, mothers formulated many theories of their own. One prominent causal ascription highlighted in this chapter involved the mother's own behavior while she was pregnant, an attribution that has been termed behavioral self-blame. Consistent with theory, mothers who made many of these self-attributions perceived more control over, and thought they could do more to prevent problems with, future pregnancies. Also highlighted was the tendency of some mothers to blame other people for this outcome. In this and previous studies, blaming others for victimizing events has almost always been associated with maladaptation. Several explanations of this relation were reviewed: (a) blaming others as a developmental diathesis, (b) the loss of personal control, (c) shattered illusions, and (d) the failure of vicarious control. Next, we turn from the analysis of mothers' appraisals of the intensive care crisis to an exploration of their deliberate efforts to cope with the stresses of their child's hospitalization.

6
Coping Strategies in the Hospital

So far, we have highlighted how mothers' appraisals of the newborn intensive care crisis can influence their well-being and predict their child's development. But appraisals that may help parents in their pursuit of meaning and mastery are not the same as their *deliberate* efforts to cope with the stresses of this event—in other words, their coping strategies. Our analysis would be incomplete if we ignore the many ways in which these parents consciously try to mitigate the stresses of their child's hospitalization. In this chapter, we summarize what we learned about the nature, determinants, and the short and longer term effects of mothers' initial coping strategies.

Our inquiry began with a global question about the things mothers did or thought to try to cope with their child's hospitalization. All mothers were able to describe at least one way in which they tried to reduce the aversiveness of this event, and most mothers more than one way. Forty-three percent of the mothers used active coping behaviors that were aimed at altering the stressful situation. In this category we included such statements as "visiting the unit every day," "contributing to the child's care," and other actions that were directed at improving the baby's health and developmentt. Just as many mothers described the importance of seeking emotional support from their spouse, other family members, and friends. Thirty percent identified information-seeking ("asking questions," "reading about the problem," "getting the facts") as one of their coping strategies. Twenty-eight percent mentioned their reliance on positive or optimistic thinking: "telling myself that things would turn out all right," "focusing on the baby's progress," and "always hoping for the best." Twenty-six percent alluded to prayer and religious devotions, such as "going to church" and "placing my faith in God." The same proportion said that they tried occasionally to distract themselves from the problem ("keeping busy with outside activities," "keeping up with my hobbies to keep my mind off my troubles"). Less commonly reported coping strategies were ventilating emotional distress (15%), finding support from parents of other babies in the NICU (12%), placing their faith in the medical staff (11%), accepting the problem (10%), and focusing on the present, as in "taking things one day at a time" (9%).

A more comprehensive, theory-guided, and quantitative analysis of mothers' coping solutions was afforded by asking them to complete the Ways of Coping Checklist, a standard questionnaire with well documented reliability and validity (Tennen & Herzberger, 1985a). Before describing this checklist and our findings, a brief review of the rationale and background of the questionnaire would be helpful.

A Definition of Coping

The work of Lazarus and Folkman supplies the most widely accepted framework for conceptualizing strategies of coping with stressful events. They view coping as "cognitive and behavorial efforts to manage external and/or internal demands that are appraised as taxing or exceeding the resources of the person" (Lazarus & Folkman, 1984, p. 141). This definition regards coping as a process that can change over the course of a threatening encounter. From this perspective, coping is what individuals think or do about a stressful problem, not how effectively they can alleviate their distress or alter the stressful situation. As such, it does not assume that certain coping strategies are more adaptive than others. The success of a coping strategy in a given situation can be determined by its relation to indicators of adjustment, such as emotional well-being, self-esteem, and daily functioning.

Lazarus and other theorists have described many overlapping taxon-omies of specific coping responses to stressful life events (Billings & Moos, 1981; Lazarus & Folkman, 1984; Pearlin & Schooler, 1978). Stone, Helder, and Schneider (1988) listed several methods of coping that are common to most formulations. These include such strategies as seeking social support, seeking information about the problem, seeking meaning in the event, taking instrumental actions to solve the problem, trying to escape the problem, and attempting to minimize the situation.

Coping and Adjustment to Stressful Events

Many investigators have been studying the ways in which people's use of these coping strategies affect their adaptation to a range of different stressful events. In this section, we illustrate what is known about the relations between adjustment and coping strategies measured by the Ways of Coping Checklist (WOCC; Lazarus & Folkman, 1984).

Items appearing in the WOCC describe a broad range of behavioral and cognitive coping strategies that might be used during a stressful encounter. Items were originally devised to sample the broad distinction between *problem-focused* strategies, aimed at changing the stressful situation, and *emotion-focused* strategies, aimed at reducing psychological disequilibrium. A series of factor analytic studies has revealed a more complex structure than is captured by this dichotomy (e.g., Coyne, Aldwin, & Lazarus, 1981; Folkman & Lazarus, 1985; Parkes, 1984; Revenson, 1981; Vingerhoets & Flohr, 1984). These other investigators have identified subscales that, although labeled differently, comprise similar items. One category involves avoidant coping, also termed withdrawal, escaping, or wishful thinking. A second category comprises attempts to find emotional support or information. A third centers on efforts to minimize the severity of the situation or to distance oneself psychologically from the problem. A fourth grouping centers on the search for meaning and has also been termed cognitive restructuring or positive reappraisal. A fifth factor involves blaming oneself or accepting responsibility for the problem. A sixth has typically been labeled planful problem-solving or taking instrumental actions.

Folkman & Lazarus (1980) initiated their research on the WOCC with a study of 100 middle-aged community residents, who described their efforts to cope with many different stresses over the course of a year. Their findings showed that both problem-focused and emotion-focused strategies were used in 98% of the stressful encounters, confirming the importance of viewing coping in terms of both problem-solving and emotion-regulation. They found as well that the context, more than the person, dictated the coping response. For example, problem-focused coping was used more often in work-related situations and emotion-focused coping was used more frequently in illness-related situations. Moreover, stressful events appraised by the person as changeable were more likely to elicit problem-focused coping, whereas events viewed as immutable more often elicited emotion-focused coping.

Most investigators using the WOCC have examined relations between coping strategies and indicators of adjustment to the stressful encounter. These studies demonstrate that the relation between coping strategies and psychological adaptation can differ according to the nature of the stressor. For example, Baum, Fleming, and Singer (1983) found that the greater use of emotion-focused coping correlated with less distress in residents who lived near the site of the Three-Mile Island disaster. Lambert (1981), in contrast, reported that the greater use of emotion-focused coping was inversely related to psychological well-being. Other studies show complex relations between adaptation and the use of specific strategies within the problem- and emotion-focused coping domains. In a study of people with one of four chronic illnesses, Felton et al. (Felton & Revenson, 1984; Felton, Revenson, & Hinrichsen, 1984) found that seeking information (a problem-focused coping strategy) and cognitive restructuring (an emotion-focused strategy) was associated with better adaptation, whereas avoidance and wishful thinking (two other categories of emotion-focused coping) were associated with poorer adaptation. Aldwin and Revenson's (1987) study of a large community sample showed that taking instrumental actions to cope with stressful events predicted less psychological distress, whereas greater use of escapist and support-seeking coping strategies predicted greater distress. Revenson & Felton (1989) found that information seeking predicted improvements in emotional well-being among individuals with rheumatoid arthritis, whereas wishful thinking predicted declines in well-being. In two other studies of rheumatoid arthritis patients (Parker et al., 1988; Manne & Zautra, 1989), wishful thinking was related to poorer adaptation and cognitive restructuring to better adaptation. Among individuals with impaired fertility (Stanton, Tennen, Affleck, & Mendola, 1990) and victims of smell loss (Tennen et al., in press), avoidant coping was also associated with greater distress.

From this diverse pattern of findings, it is difficult to predict which coping strategies may be adaptive or maladaptive for mothers of infants hospitalized on a NICU. However, there is some consensus from previous research using the WOCC that escapist/avoidant coping strategies are associated with greater psychological distress, whereas cognitive restructuring/ positive appraisal strategies are connected with psychological well-being.

Descriptive Findings

At NICU discharge, mothers replied, on 4-point scales, how much they had used each of the WOCC's 66 coping strategies as a way of coping with the hospital crisis. Among the many scoring approaches for this checklist available in the literature, we adopted the procedure used by Aldwin and Revenson (1987) in their large community sample of adults. We evaluated the internal consistencies of each of their factor scores in our sample and incorporated in our analyses only those coping factor scores whose alpha coefficients were greater than .60. Those meeting this criterion have emerged most frequently in factor analytic studies of the WOCC. The specific factors, the number of items in each factor, and examples of items comprising each factor are as follows:

Taking Instrumental Actions (seven items): "I made a plan of action and followed it"; "I came up with a couple of different solutions to the problem"

Mobilizing Social Support (six items): "Talked to someone to find out more about the situation"; "I asked a relative or friend I respected for advice"

Seeking Meaning (four items): "I tried to discover new faith or some important truth"; "I tried to discover what is important in life"

Escaping (seven items): "I had fantasies or wishes about how things might turn out"; "I wished that the situation would go away or somehow be over with"; "I thought about fantastic or unreal things that made me feel better"

Minimizing (nine items): "I went on as if nothing happened"; "I tried to accept and make the best of it"; "I made light of the situation and refused to get too serious about it"

Scores for items within each of the coping factors were summed and divided by the number of items to allow comparison across coping strategies. Then, we followed the computational procedure recommended by Vitaliano, Maiuro, Russo, & Becker (1985) to create relative coping scores, that is, scores that reflect the relative importance of each coping strategy in a mother's overall distribution of coping efforts. This scheme controls for differences in the amount of coping that has occurred during the encounter, capturing instead the pattern of coping strategies. Each coping score could range from 0, indicating no use of that coping strategy, to 1, indicating the exclusive use of that coping strategy.

The distribution of the five coping strategies within our sample is portrayed in Figure 6.1 The most commonly used coping strategies by mothers in this situation were seeking meaning and mobilizing social support. Most mothers used a combination of coping strategies, in varying degrees. There were no mothers who did not minimize to some extent, one mother who did not seek support, one who did not take instrumental actions, one who did not seek meaning, and two who did not try to escape from the problem, however slightly.

Correlates of Coping Strategies

Our next aim was to examine some of the correlates of mothers' use of these coping strategies. The younger mothers and the mothers of first-borns used escapist coping to a significantly greater extent. Mothers who had other children were more apt to take instrumental actions to cope with the intensive care crisis. Mothers who used more escapist coping reported less positive mood at discharge, and those who tried to minimize the problem reported more positive mood (see Table 6.1), even when background variables were controlled statistically. Thus, mothers who

FIGURE 6.1. Distribution of mothers' relative coping strategies as measured by the Ways of Coping Checklist (WOCC).

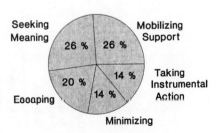

TABLE 6.1. Relations of in-hospital coping strategies to mothers' and children's outcomes.

Outcome	Coping strategy				
	Instrumental action	Mobilizing support	Minimizing	Escaping	Seeking meaning
At discharge					
Positive mood	.03	−.08	.22*	−.31**	.16
At 6 mos.					
Positive mood	.08	.11	.04	−.24**	.01
Depression	−.02	−.07	−.06	.21*	−.07
Attachment	.03	.06	−.08	−.12	.10
Competence	.13	.08	−.03	−.17	−.01
Responsiveness	−.10	.12	.01	−.02	−.02
At 18 mos.					
Positive mood	−.22*	.07	.17	−.18	.12
Global distress	.24*	−.05	−.18	.15	−.34**
Home environment	.22*	.15	.12	−.24*	.09
Developmental outcome	.07	−.18	.00	−.13	.25*

* $p < .05$.
** $p < .01$.

tried to escape from the problem may have done so because of their younger age, the fact that this was their first-born child, and perhaps because they were experiencing more emotional distress. Their greater emotional distress could also be because of the relative ineffectiveness of escapist coping strategies as a way of alleviating distress (Aldwin & Revenson, 1987).

In Chapter 1, we depicted the many different stresses comprising the crisis of newborn intensive care. The coping strategies of mothers who described some of the more common stresses were compared with those of mothers who did not report these challenges. Specifically, we determined if mothers coped differently when they did or did not mention the denial of care, the infant's uncertain survival, the technological environment of the NICU, or the baby's suffering as a key feature of the intensive care crisis. To summarize these findings, mothers who described the crisis as involving the denial of their caregiving responsibilities were more apt to cope by escaping and less likely to cope through taking instrumental actions. Second, those mothers who mentioned the technological aspects of the NICU as one of the more difficult problems with which they had to cope were also more likely to cope through escapist strategies. Third, those mothers who mentioned their infant's uncertain survival as a major challenge were less likely to minimize the severity of the situation. Last, mothers who commented on the baby's suffering in describing the challenges of the intensive care crisis were more apt to seek support as a way of coping with the hospitalization.

Coping Predictors of Mother and Child Outcomes

A more powerful demonstration of the effect of coping strategies on parents' well-being and behavioral adaptation is afforded by their ability to predict mothers' adaptational outcomes 6 and 18 months after discharge. First, we examined how each of the coping strategies reported at NICU discharge might predict how mothers were faring 6 months later. As Table 6.1 indicates, the only coping strategy that predicted 6-month outcomes was escapist coping. Those who used this strategy to a greater extent became more depressed and had less positive mood at 6 months. However, when background variables and mothers' mood at discharge were taken into account, neither of these relations remained significant, primarily because of the concurrent association of this coping strategy with mood disturbance.

A different picture emerged from our analyses of the predictive significance of mothers' coping strategies for mothers' and children's longer term outcomes assessed 18 months after discharge (see Table 6.1). Mothers whose coping with newborn intensive care had been characterized by taking more instrumental actions reported more symptoms of psychological distress and less positive mood. At the same time, these mothers were providing more optimal home environments for their developing child. On the other hand, mothers whose coping had been characterized by more escaping provided less optimal support to their child's development. Mothers who were experiencing fewer symptoms of psychological distress at 18 months were more likely to have coped with their child's hospitalization by trying to find meaning in the experience. Finally, the only coping strategy that predicted the child's developmental status was seeking meaning: mothers using this strategy more had children who exhibited superior development 18 months later.

The specificity of early coping strategies as predictors of mothers' and children's outcomes 18 months after discharge was examined through hierarchical regression models in which a block of background variables and mothers' mood at NICU discharge was entered first in the equations. Then, each of the five coping strategies was entered to determine if it still accounted for additional variation in the 18-month outcomes. These analyses showed that taking instrumental actions remained a predictor of both greater global psychological distress and less positive mood, but more optimal home environments, and that seeking meaning still predicted better developmental outcomes for the child.

In our last set of analyses we determined whether the long-term effect of mothers' strategies of coping with newborn intensive care might depend on the child's developmental outcome. To answer this question, we constructed another set of hierarchical regression equations. As before, we first entered the block of variables measured at NICU discharge. Then, the presence or absence of a developmental disability at 18 months was forced into the equation. Coping strategies were entered next, in separate equations. Then, the effect of coping strategies, conditional upon the presence or absence of a disability, was captured in the final set of interaction terms entered in the equations.

The regression equations predicting mothers' mood and global distress and the quality of the home environment yielded several significant interactions, indicating that the relation between early coping strategies and these outcomes differed depending on the child's developmental outcome, that is, the presence or absence of a developmental disability at 18 months. Three significant interactions were found for the prediction of mothers' mood: the mobilizing support by developmental disability interaction, taking instrumental actions by disability interaction, and seeking meaning by disability interaction. The nature of these interactions is portrayed in Figure 6.2, which expresses the specific relations between coping strategies at NICU discharge and mothers' mood at 18 months for two groups of mothers: those whose child had a normal outcome and those whose child was developmentally disabled. To summarize, seeking meaning and mobilizing support predicted more positive mood for mothers whose child had a subsequent developmental disability, but did not predict mood for mothers whose child had a normal outcome.

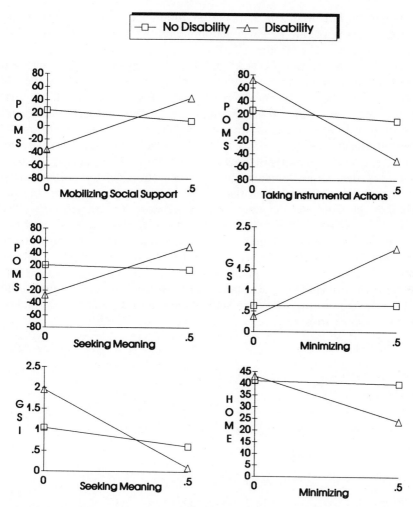

FIGURE 6.2. Predictive significance of mothers' coping strategies as a function of the presence or absence of a developmental disability at 18 months.

Two interactions were significant predictors of mothers' symptoms of psychological distress: the minimizing by disability interaction and the seeking meaning by disability interaction. As is shown in Figure 6.2, mothers who had done more minimizing became more distressed only when their child's outcome was poor. And seeking meaning was a stronger predictor of freedom from distress for mothers whose child was developmentally disabled than for those with a normally developing child. Finally, the prediction of HOME Inventory scores afforded by minimizing the problem also depended on the presence or absence of a disability. As Figure 6.2 shows, when the child's outcome was normal, minimizing the problem did not predict later home environments. But when the child's outcome was poor, mothers who had done more minimizing provided less optimal home environments.

The hospitalization of a newborn on an intensive care unit elicits a spectrum of coping strategies summarized in this chapter. They include efforts to act directly on the source of the stress, to seek social support, pursue meaning in the crisis, minimize the severity of the problem, and escape or withdraw from the situation. We showed that the use of some of these strategies not only predicted differences in how mothers were feeling a year and a half later but also how well their child was developing. In some instances, the predictive significance of coping strategies for mothers' long-term well-being depended on the nature of the child's outcome, that is, whether the child was diagnosed as developmentally disabled.

With the close of this chapter, we end our analysis of how mothers' intrapersonal resources—their search for meaning, mastery, and causes and their use of coping strategies—aided their adaptation to their child's intensive care and its aftermath. In the next chapter, we broaden our framework to include the adaptational benefits of mothers' interpersonal resources—their interactions with family and friends, and their ability to obtain support from the staff of the intensive care unit.

7
The Search for Social Support

As we demonstrated in Chapter 6, mothers often seek support from others as a way of coping with newborn intensive care. Their need for support can sometimes be met by professionals, but appropriate supportive services are not always available. Thus, parents may need to rely heavily on their informal support network, securing help from their spouse, other relatives, and friends. Unfortunately, whereas the birth of a healthy child usually stimulates social contact and increases opportunities for support (Belsky, 1983), the birth of a sick or premature infant may reduce parents' usual level of support, and worse, may disrupt close interpersonal relationships (Zarling, Hirsch, & Landry, 1988). The theme of this chapter is how other people figure in parents' ability to adapt to the hospitalization and home-coming of medically fragile infants. We analyze how mothers' satisfaction with support providers, need for support, interpersonal conflicts, and social isolation contributed to their adaptation.

The Benefits of Social Support

Social support is a multidimensional construct, with affective, cognitive, and instrumental elements. A wide range of needs can be met by social support, including intimate interaction, advice, information, and tangible aid (Barrera, 1981; Cohen & McKay, 1984). Support may also help restore cherished beliefs that are threatened by victimization. As Janoff-Bulman (1989) observes, "the presence of caring, supportive others provides direct evidence of benevolence in the world, of people responding when one needs them, and of one's self-worth" (p. 166).

There is substantial evidence that social support buffers the impact of stressful life events and chronic stressors. Support to new parents has been shown to influence their child-rearing behavior and attitudes, including their sense of competence and feelings of self-efficacy (Abernathy, 1973;

Cutrona & Troutman, 1986; Sirigano, Kozinn, & Lachman, 1987), their responsiveness to the child (Crnic, Greenberg, Robinson, & Ragozin, 1984; Garcia-Coll, 1983), and their provision of optimal home environments for a developing child (Crnic, Greenberg, & Slough, 1986; Pascoe, Loda, Jeffries, & Earp, 1981). Social support has also been linked to adjustment among parents of young children with special needs (Affleck et al., 1986; Crnic, Greenberg, Ragozin, Robinson, & Basham, 1983; Dunst & Trivette, 1987; Dunst, Trivette, & Cross, 1985; Gowan, Appelbaum, & Johnson-Martin, 1987; Trause & Kramer, 1983).

Shumaker and Brownell (1984) define social support as the provision of resources that are "perceived by the provider or the recipient to be intended to enhance the well-being of the recipient" (p. 13). From this perspective, parents' perceptions of the helpfulness or unhelpfulness of support providers' behavior need to be considered to achieve a fuller understanding of the support process. Recent investigations of individuals with rheumatoid arthritis (Affleck, Pfeiffer, et al., 1988), parents of children with cancer (Chesler & Barbarin, 1984), and people who have lost a loved one in an accident (Lehman, Ellard, & Wortman, 1986) reveal how even well-meaning support gestures can constitute an additional source of strain. Help-giving, especially when it is unsolicited or unnecessary, can even be harmful when it undermines the recipient's self-esteem and sense of mastery (Chesler & Barbarin, 1984; Revenson, Wollman, & Felton, 1983). Brickman, Rabinowitz, Karuza, Coates, Cohn, & Kidder (1982) note that awkward or ineffective support to people in crisis can even create a process of "secondary victimization."

Our research with individuals with rheumatoid arthritis illustrates some of the complexities of the relation between social support and adjustment to threatening circumstances (Affleck, Pfeiffer, et al., 1988). These individuals were asked to rate their satisfaction with social support in several areas comprising informational, emotional, and tangible support. Independent of sociodemographic factors and the severity of their illness, those who were more satisfied with their support in these areas were rated by their care providers as exhibiting superior psychological adjustment. We offered several interpretations of this finding. First, a satisfying network of supportive relationships can represent an important resource for people who are contending with life stresses and strains. A second possibility is that individuals who are adjusting less well to their illness might find it more difficult to attract and maintain support. A third explanation is that those who are adjusting less well have greater expectations of their support network. Accordingly, they may be relatively less satisfied with levels of support that others with fewer expectations would find acceptable. We also demonstrated a "stress-buffering" role of social support inasmuch as the support-adjustment relation was stronger for individuals who were more disabled by their illness.

Appraisals of Support During the Hospitalization

Support Satisfaction

In a study of another sample of mothers of medically fragile infants, we showed that satisfaction with support during the first weeks after NICU discharge was unrelated to the amount of support mothers were receiving (Affleck et al., 1986). We also found that evaluations of support, not the frequency of support, figured in their adjustment.

Mothers' answers to four questions on the Arizona Social Support Questionnaire (Barrera, 1981) provided an index of their satisfaction with the support they had obtained from others during their child's hospitalization. On 3-point scales, they rated their satisfaction with "opportunities to talk to people about personal and private feelings," "obtaining physical help and material aid from others," "obtaining feedback from others," and "obtaining advice from others." The mean score on this measure (which could range from 4 to 12) was 10.01, indicating that most mothers were generally satisfied with the support they had been able to secure from others during their child's stay on the intensive care unit.

In addition to offering these global appraisals of support satisfaction, mothers used a 5-point scale to record their satisfaction with each of seven potential support providers. In rank order of satisfaction, these were (a) the baby's father (mean = 4.54); (b) the baby's primary nurse (mean = 4.52); (c) their own mother (mean = 4.24); (d) their best friend (mean = 3.82); (e) their child's physicians (mean = 3.75); (f) any siblings (mean = 3.73); and (g) their own father (mean = 3.54).

Each mother was also asked to consider the ways in which she had been helped by the individual who, all things considered, gave her the most support during her child's hospitalization. She read a list of statements describing eight of these support functions and recorded her agreement with each on a 5-point scale. Table 7.1 lists the results. Mothers' primary support providers helped them most by helping them to maintain their self-esteem, to see the situation in a better light, and to accept the situation.

TABLE 7.1. Support functions met by mothers' primary support provider.

Function	Mean	% Strongly agree
Helping me feel good about myself	4.50	65.0
Helping me see the situation in a better light	4.33	53.3
Helping me to accept the situation	4.33	44.8
Helping me to take my mind off things	4.28	49.5
Allowing me to express my feelings	4.27	57.1
Making things easier for me to spend time with my baby	4.21	60.6
Giving me advice on how to help my baby	3.90	44.8
Giving me information about the problem	3.77	41.0

The need for information and advice was not as readily met, probably because more than 80% of the mothers identified the baby's father as the primary support provider.

Mothers' global satisfaction with support was not affected by their age, education, parity, or the severity of their infant's medical problems. More satisfied mothers, however, did report more positive mood at NICU discharge ($r = .21, p < .05$). Considering mothers' satisfaction with their individual support providers, mothers of first-born infants were more pleased with their husband's support, and mothers with more education were more pleased with both their husband's and their best friend's support. Mothers who were more satisfied with the physician's support expressed more positive mood at discharge ($r = .23, p < .05$).

The absence of significant relations between mothers' emotional well-being and their satisfaction with other support providers' behavior should not be construed as evidence that these individuals played no part in mothers' adaptation. Rather, this may reflect the fact that few mothers were dissatisfied with the help they received from some of these individuals. For example, only rarely were mothers displeased with the support they received from their child's father or their child's primary nurse. We suspect that the withdrawal of these important sources of support would have been a great loss. Many mothers, including the woman quoted next, described the solace they could derive only from their spouse:

> Sometimes after coming home from the hospital, we would just lie in bed and cry together. It was like we were the only people in the world who were going through this. After that, we would talk openly about our feelings, and that's how we got through it. I found it difficult to do this with my parents and friends because I didn't want them to be upset.

In reviewing the interview transcripts, we found few critical comments about the support mothers were able to find from the NICU nursing staff. Occasionally, a mother would single out a nurse as being "uncaring and insensitive" but would usually qualify her remarks about this individual as standing in contrast to the rest of the nursing staff. The appreciation many mothers felt for the support they received from their child's nurse is typified by the following comment:

> The thing I remember most was how the nurses in the unit were so supportive. They would go out of their way to answer all my questions. If I had opinions, they'd listen to these. As bad as it was, they really made me feel at home and gave me everything my child and I needed. Without their help, I don't see how I could ever have handled this.

The complex relations between people's adjustment to aversive life events and their ability to obtain support (Coyne & DeLongis, 1986) must be considered in order to intepret the relation between support satisfaction and emotional adaptation. For example, mothers who encountered problems in obtaining support from their child's physician may well be placed at a disadvantage. But those who are more distressed could also want more from the treatment staff, accounting for their relative displeasure with what they obtained. What's more, physicians may have avoided contact with parents who were more distressed. Support may aid adjustment, but people who are contending less well with a crisis may find it harder to attract and maintain support from others (Silver & Wortman, 1980). Thus, relations between well-being and support satisfaction are probably reciprocal.

Mothers' Perceptions of Helpful and Unhelpful Support

We also asked mothers to descibe "the things that people did or said that were helpful in your efforts to cope with this crisis" and "what people said or did that added further strain to your efforts to cope." Response categories and their proportions are presented in Table 7.2

The most helpful support gestures involved expressions of concern and caring, providing reassurance about their coping abilities, and tangible aid when needed. Expressions of concern and caring ranged from simply acknowledging the baby's birth by sending cards to actually accompanying parents to the hospital. Many parents were grateful to hear from friends and relatives that "they would be there if we needed someone to talk to." The importance of this gesture echoes findings from studies of other stressful events (Affleck, Pfeiffer et al., 1988; Dunkel-Schetter, 1984; Lehman et al., 1986). Apparently the opportunity to ventilate feelings and concerns is a valued resource for people in crisis. Several mothers also appreciated others' efforts to reassure them about their coping abilities, as in "being told by nurses that I was doing so well," "hearing that I have the strength to pull me through this crisis," and "pointing out how what I was doing was helping my baby." Some were also relieved to hear that their painful feelings were normal in this situation. Gestures involving tangible aid consisted largely of efforts to make things easier for mothers to spend

TABLE 7.2. Mothers' appraisals of helpful and unhelpful support gestures.

	Percent	
Category	Helpful	Unhelpful
Expressions of concern and caring	42.5	0.0
Reassurance about own coping abilities	26.5	0.0
Optimistic statements about child	24.8	7.1
Providing tangible support	22.1	0.0
Emphasizing positive outcomes for similar children	15.0	7.1
Encouraging a philosophical perspective	7.1	7.1
Insensitive remarks	0.0	21.2
Pessimistic statements about child	0.0	15.0
Being blamed for the problem	0.0	6.2
Family and friends withdrawing	0.0	13.3

time with the baby in the hospital (e.g., baby sitting, cooking meals).

At the same time, 63% of the mothers described how other people, even close family and friends, said or did unhelpful things. Some of the comments mothers attributed to others were viewed as insensitive, even cruel:

> Someone asked me if it was too late to change the baby's name.

> A friend said she would wait to buy a gift for the baby when it was certain he'd make it.

> My mother said how lucky I was that I wouldn't have to get up for 2 a.m. feedings.

> My sister said that I was fortunate that I had time to recover from the delivery without having to take care of a baby.

Pessimistic views about the child were never appreciated. Examples of these statements were "being prepared for the possibility that she wouldn't make it," and "hearing stories about similar babies who died." Finally, several mothers remarked how some of their closest friends and relatives "seemed to always find an excuse to avoid us," "never really acknowledged the baby's birth," or simply "stopped calling."

A key finding is that some of the same support gestures viewed by some parents as helpful were seen by others as harmful. For example, whereas several mothers said they appreciated hearing optimistic statements about their child's future, a few were offended by others' attempts to paint a rosy picture of the outcome. They were troubled by what they saw as the encouragement of "false hope." One mother told us why this was unhelpful:

> My mother kept telling us not to worry, that everything would turn out all right. But she didn't have any idea what was going on. He was on his death bed. They had given him the last rights. I didn't want anyone telling me that he was going to be fine. It would just lift my hopes too much. If I believed this, and he did die, I would die too in a way.

In a similar vein, some mothers said they were uplifted by stories about other sick or premature infants who survived without any future problems. In one mother's opinion, "It was good to hear that there was a light at the end of the tunnel, that babies like mine can turn out all right." But others were upset by similar stories, stating, as one mother did, that "they just didn't appreciate how unique our situation was... that you just couldn't compare our child with any other." Finally, several mothers said they benefited from others' encouragement of a philosophical perspective, as in being reminded "to trust in God's will," "that we were privileged to give birth to a needy child," or "to look on the bright side of this experience." Yet, others resisted these attempts to promote a positive interpretation of this experience. As one mother exclaimed,

My sister is forever reminding me that things could have been worse... that my baby could have died. But I can't get over the thought that things could have turned out better, that this shouldn't have happened at all!

Relatives and friends were mentioned more frequently than were health professionals as the sources of unhelpful support. One reason why intimate support providers may not always be helpful is that they may have an overriding interest in seeing the victim recover quickly from the crisis (Lehman et al., 1986). This can lead to expectations of a premature recovery and the discouragement of expressions of concern, doubt, and painful feelings.

Mothers who reported any unhelpful support gestures were significantly less satisfied with the support they had obtained during their child's hospitalization. But they also said they needed more support from others. This substantiates our impression that many mothers who criticized others' helping efforts seemed to hold greater expectations of these individuals. Hence, before summarizing findings on mothers' social network characteristics and their relations to mothers' well-being and adaptation after NICU discharge, we will enumerate the determinants and possible consequences of mothers' differing need for support during their child's hospitalization and after 6 months of caring for their child at home.

The Need for Support

People differ in how much they need support during stressful times, and their needs may frame their satisfaction with the support they actually receive. Moreover, mothers whose infants had more severe medical problems and those who were more distressed may well have needed more support. Thus, any relation between support satisfaction and adjustment could be due to mothers' differing need for support.

At hospital discharge, and again 6 months later, mothers' answers to four questions on the Arizona Social Support Questionnaire (Barrera, 1981) provided an index of their need for social support. On 3-point scales, they rated their need for "opportunities to talk to people about personal and private feelings," "obtaining physical help and material aid from others," "obtaining feedback from others," and "obtaining advice from others." With possible scores ranging from 4 to 12, the average need for support score before discharge was 8.77 and six months after discharge was 7.59. Mothers needing more support before discharge tended to be those who needed more support after discharge. But as a group, their need for support while their baby was hospitalized was greater than what they felt after they took their baby home.

Mothers' need for support during their child's hospitalization was not a function of situational variables: mothers needing more support did not differ on major background characteristics nor was their child's medical condition any more severe. But they did report more emotional distress at NICU discharge ($r = -.21$, $p < .05$). Similarly, mothers who said they needed more support after NICU discharge scored lower on measures of their emotional well-being and adaptation, including reports of less positive mood ($r = -.30$, $p < .01$), more depression ($r = .39$, $p < .01$), less attachment to the child ($r = -.32$, $p < .01$), and less perceived competence ($r = -.53$, $p < .01$).

During the hospitalization and period of the transition home, mothers needing more support were less satisfied with the support they received. To determine whether any concurrent relations between support satisfaction and well-being might be explained by mothers' need for support, the latter variable was controlled statistically. This procedure showed that the relation between mothers' support satisfaction and positive mood before NICU discharge was attributable to the greater need for support among the more distressed mothers. However, most of the concurrent relations between support satisfaction and adaptation at 6 months (see Table 7.3) were not affected by controlling for mothers' need for support after discharge. Thus, the link between mothers' evaluation of their social support and their adjustment after discharge was not because mothers needing more support were both less satisfied with their support and faring less well.

Further analyses showed that mothers needing more support before and after hospital discharge were less satisfied with their support regardless of their emotional well-being at either time. Thus, even though adaptational problems might increase mothers' need for support, our findings indicate that the relation between need for support and satisfaction with support is not accounted for by these problems. Perhaps mothers needing more support simply had greater expectations of their support network and were more likely to be disappointed by others' ability to help.

Appraisals of Support After Discharge

Support Satisfaction and Amount of Support

Mothers were more satisfied with the support they were finding after discharge than with the support they had found before discharge. But the absence of a relation between support satisfaction before and after discharge suggests that some mothers who had found satisfying levels of support when their child was in the hospital did not do so during the transition home, and vice versa. Thus, there may be an inconsistent response from mothers' social network across the phases of this crisis, or again, mothers' expectations of their support network may change across time. Mothers who actually obtained more support during the transition home (as measured by the Inventory of Socially Supportive Behaviors) did not express greater satisfaction with their support, indicating that mothers' satisfaction with their support network does not depend on the frequency with which support was provided.

Interpersonal Conflict and Social Isolation

Previous research shows that conflicts with support providers play a unique role in people's adjustment to stressful life events and are unrelated to the support these individuals provide (Barrera, 1981; Fiore, Becker, & Coppel, 1983; Rook, 1984). In a study of mothers of typical infants, difficult encounters with social network members were intensified by problems in the child's development (Parks & Lenz, 1987). As we noted in Chapter 1, many mothers found that conflicts with family and friends were among the most difficult problems they faced during the transition from hospital to home care. One of the more disturbing consequences of a lack of support may be that mothers find themselves isolated from social contacts.

After caring for their child at home for six months, mothers were asked about the number of individuals with whom they had conflicts concerning their child. As predicted, the size of the conflicted network was unrelated to mothers' satisfaction with social support, suggesting that support providers can be both helpful and harmful in their interactions with these mothers. Mothers who reported greater social isolation on the Parenting Stress Index were less satisfied with the support they had obtained. But again, feelings of social isolation had little to do with the amount of support mothers reported having received.

Social Network Correlates of Adaptation at 6 Months

Each of the four major social network variables measured at 6 months— support satisfaction, amount of support, conflicted network size, and social isolation—as well as mothers' satisfaction with support in the hospital, was inspected as a correlate of mothers' well-being and adaptation during the transition home. As Table 7.3 shows, the highest correlations with mothers' adaptation at 6 months involved social isolation: mothers reporting more isolation were not only more likely to report deficits in well-being, but were also less responsive to their child. Also, mothers' satisfaction with support, but not the amount of support they were receiving, figured in their well-being.

When background variables and mothers' mood at discharge were taken into account, significant relations remained between social support variables and mothers' adaptation. Mothers who were more satisfied with their support in the hospital reported less depression and greater attachment 6

TABLE 7.3. Relations of social network variables to mothers' and childrens' outcomes.

Variable	At 6 mos					At 18 mos			
	Positive mood	Depression	Attachment	Competence	Responsiveness	Positive mood	Global distress	HOME Inventory	Developmental outcome
At NICU discharge									
Support satisfaction	.16	-.34**	.26*	.17	.10	.18	-.27**	.19	-.08
At 6 mos									
Support satisfaction	.37**	-.36**	.35**	.49**	.14	.25*	-.22*	-.07	-.08
Amount of support	.15	.09	.04	.03	-.05	.09	-.03	.11	.02
Social isolation	-.53**	.55**	-.41**	-.48**	-.25*	-.31**	.18	-.25*	-.22*
Conflicted network size	-.34*	.11	.08	-.18	.01	-.21*	.23*	-.02	.14

* $p < .05$.
** $p < .01$.

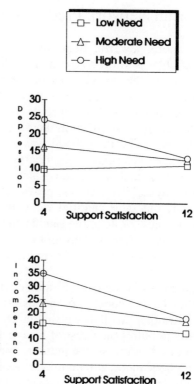

FIGURE 7.1. Relation of mothers' support satisfaction with depression and sense of incompetence as a function of need for support 6 months after discharge.

months after discharge. Satisfaction with support at 6 months remained a significant correlate of positive mood, less depression, greater attachment, and greater perceived competence. Social isolation remained a correlate of less positive mood, more depression, less attachment, and greater competence. Finally, mothers with a more conflicted social network described their mood as less positive.

An additional question is whether mothers' satisfaction with support is more critical when they feel a stronger need for support. Perhaps the adaptational problems evidenced by mothers with a high need for support can be reduced by obtaining the support they need. This was addressed by examining the interaction of support need and support satisfaction in regression equations predicting mothers' outcomes at 6 months. The satisfaction by need interaction played a role in two outcomes: depression and sense of competence. Figure 7.1 shows that support satisfaction made an even greater difference in the well-being of mothers who needed the most support. When the neediest mothers were able to obtain satisfying levels of support in the months after discharge, they were no more depressed or lacking in competence than their less needy counterparts.

Social Network Predictors of 18-Month Outcomes

A more powerful demonstration of the importance of social network variables is afforded by their prediction of 18-month outcomes. Table 7.3 presents the correlations between major social network variables and mothers' and children's outcomes a year or 18 months later. Mothers' support satisfaction before discharge predicted greater global distress, as did support satisfaction and the size of the conflicted network after discharge. Positive mood was predicted by three of the social network variables measured at six months: support satisfaction, fewer interpersonal conflicts, and less social isolation. Finally, the mothers who felt more socially isolated not only provided less optimal home environments a year later, but their children went on to exhibit less positive developmental outcomes. None of the significant relations appearing in this table held up, however, when background variables and mothers' concurrent mood were controlled statistically in multiple regression equations. Thus, we cannot infer that support characteristics alone influence mothers' and children's outcomes in the overall sample. Instead, they may be influential because they have a contemporaneous effect on mothers' well-being.

Another possibility is that mothers' satisfaction with their social support acts to buffer the stress of having a child whose developmental outcome is poor. A regression equation, controlling for background variables and mothers' mood at 6 months, revealed that mothers' satisfaction with social support at 6 months predicted their mood at 18 months only when the presence or absence of a developmental disability was taken into account. The direction of this interaction, portrayed in Figure 7.2, indicates that mothers' support satisfaction during the transition home predicted their later emotional well-being when their child was diagnosed as having a developmental disability.

Coping Strategies and Support

A final issue was anticipated in a study by Dunkel-Schetter, Folkman, and Lazarus (1987). They hypothesized that the support people receive during stressful encounters depends on their ways of coping with the event. Coping strategies may "provide cues to members of the social network regarding the person's needs and desires for support. . .and make it easy or difficult in subtle ways for others to provide support" (p. 78). They confirmed that the amount of support people obtain during a crisis increases when their coping is characterized by more problem-solving activities, efforts to seek support, and attempts to find meaning. Efforts to minimize or distance oneself from the problem were associated with less support.

To examine this question, we inspected the correlations between

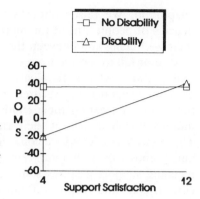

FIGURE 7.2. Predictive significance of mothers' support satisfaction at 6 months for mothers' mood at 18 months as a function of the presence or absence of a developmental disability.

mothers' strategies of coping with their child's hospitalization (see Chapter 6) and the amount of informational, emotional, and material support they reported receiving during the 6 months after dischage. Mothers who tried harder to mobilize support found it in all areas. Those who used more instrumental coping strategies received more information and advice, but not more emotional or tangible support. And, those who tried harder to minimize the problem were the recipients of less overall support.

Our findings reflect a match between mothers' coping strategies and the support they obtained. The mother who is coping by trying to mobilize support may be conveying a general need for support that others recognize and attempt to fill in a variety of ways. In contrast, the mother who is minimizing the severity of the problem may be signaling to others that support is not needed. This interpretation is strengthened by the fact that mothers who had sought more support felt a greater need for support after discharge, whereas those who had tried to minimize the problem had less of a need for support. The association between instrumental action coping and the receipt of more advice and information appears a more specific fit between coping and support. The mother who adopts this coping strategy may be especially receptive to advice and information on how to solve problems related to her child's care and could be communicating this interest to her family and friends. Our analyses do not preclude the possibility that mothers' coping strategies were themselves shaped by the support they received from others during their child's hospitalization. For example, the information and advice that mothers receive from others may encourage the pursuit of problem-directed solutions. Hence, the coping-support relation is best conceptualized as one that involves nonrecursive processes and mutual influence (Dunkel-Schetter et al., 1987)

This chapter focused on the role of other people in parents' ability to adapt to the hospitalization and homecoming of medically fragile infants. We documented how mothers' satisfaction with support providers, need for support, interpersonal conflicts, and social isolation contributed to their adaptation. We raised important issues about the complex interdependencies of people's need for support, their satisfaction with support, and their well-being and between their coping strategies and the support they receive or fail to receive from others. One interpretation of our findings is that mothers who were pleased with the assistance, information, and emotional support they secured from their family, friends, and the health professionals treating their child were better able to contend with the multifaceted demands of their child's hospitalization and its aftermath. These mothers offered welcome insights into the ways in which relatives and friends can be helpful. Yet most mothers also described how well-meaning support gestures sometimes did more harm than good or how close friends and relatives distanced themselves.

Most of the married mothers praised the support they had obtained from their husband, and most named their husband as the one person who gave them the greatest help and comfort. In particular, husbands were able to help their wife maintain her self-esteem during this crisis. In Chapter 9, we will examine in greater detail the mutual support that is available within the martial relationship. Before doing so, we explore in the next chapter the importance of social support, coping strategies, and cognitive adaptations in mothers' active memories of their child's hospitalization during the first and second years after hospital discharge.

8
Mothers' Remembrances of Newborn Intensive Care

A compelling reason why a newborn's intensive care can have a lasting effect on parents' psychological well-being is that they re-experience this event in memory. Some of the participants in our study, including the mothers quoted next, volunteered that the distress ensuing from their memories even exceeded that which they had felt during theirr child's hospitalization itself.

> The emotional trauma of having your child in an ICU gets even worse after you leave it behind. When it's happening, nobody gives you a choice, nobody asks you if you can handle it or not. When you get home, and begin the remember it, that's when it hits you. . . the full awareness that she had just as much a chance of dying as living.

> When you're in the unit, you believe everything they say to try to keep your spirits up. You get wound up in how many breaths a minute they're taking, how much air is pumped in and out. You get absorbed in the numbers and the machines. But when you come home, and you start to remember all of this, you start realizing how chancy everything was, and that is very, very scary.

> At the time, we were caught up in pulling for her to live and the business of the treatment. Now, with all that behind us, the emotional impact hits me when I find myself remembering that time.

> My memories are upsetting me, because with time I've had a chance to digest just how bad the situation was. I wonder how I was ever able to make it through that time.

Years after other losses or traumatic events, many people describe vivid memories of the acute crisis (Lehman, Wortman, & Williams, 1987; Silver, Boon, & Stones, 1983). For these individuals, environmental cues act as reminders that keep the distressing event from settling into the past (Silver et al., 1983; Spinetta, Swarner, & Sheposh, 1981). This "reliving" of stressful experiences may account, in part, for the prolonged psychological recovery from victimization (Silver & Wortman, 1980). From another perspective, the persistence of these memories can signal continuing efforts to master the threatening event (Horowitz, 1983) or to find its meaning

(Silver et al., 1983). What is not resolved at the time of the event's occurrence may well remain with the victim as part of his long-term memory and intrude in day-to-day life.

Gunn, Lepore, and Outerbridge (1983) found that most mothers continue to have distressing memories years after their child has been discharged from a NICU. Some had recurring nightmares and found themselves re-experiencing the anxieties associated with their child's hospitalization. In a study of another group of mothers (Affleck, Tennen et al., 1985; Affleck et al., 1986) we showed that those who were having more intrusive memories of the hospitalization and were attempting to avoid reminders of it were more emotionally distressed and less satisfied with their infant. The cross-sectional design of these studies and the lack of descriptive information on the content, emotional range, and environmental triggers of mothers' memories limit interpretation and understanding of this phenomenon. In this chapter, we present more detailed, longitudinal findings concerning the memories mothers had after they took their child home from the hospital. We also extend our earlier study of mothers' intrusive thoughts and avoidance of reminders into the second year after discharge.

Memories of the Hospitalization

Our first objective was to document individual differences in the content and emotional character of mothers' recurring memories. We expected that many of the stressful features of the crisis discussed in Chapter 1 would be featured in mothers' remembrances, including feelings of helplessness, the infant's uncertain survival, the novel and chaotic intensive care environment, and difficulties in obtaining needed support. At the same time, as we demonstrated in Chapters 3 and 4, many mothers find benefits and meaning in their misfortune, cherish the support they were able to obtain from others while their infant was in the NICU, and are uplifted by the child's survival "against the odds." Thus, we reasoned that some mothers might also find themselves recalling favorable characteristics of their child's hospitalization. We can make no claim that mothers' memories of specific events occurring in the hospital are veridical. Work on autobiographical memory (Vaillant, 1977; Woodruff & Brien, 1972) demonstrates that people do not always accurately recall their life experiences. Rather, they often reconstruct those events to suit current needs and to maintain an integrated, usually benevolent, view of themselves. Similarly, parents' memories of the hospitalization may be distortions of actual events or even inventions.

In both the 6- and 18-month follow-up interviews, mothers were asked: "During the past month have you been experiencing any memories of your child's hospitalization on the newborn intensive care unit; that is do you still find yourself remembering or reminiscing about the time when your child was in the hospital?" Five mothers who were asked this question at 6 months replied that they had experienced no memories in the past month, and three reported no recent memories at 18 months. These few mothers were intent on turning away from the experience:

> The day he came home from the hospital, I was determined that we were just going to move ahead and put this experience behind us. I don't even have to try to block it out now. It just doesn't play a role in my life anymore. There's so much happening now, I don't have the time to play remember when.

> I just refuse to let myself think about that time. I had to, or else I would become depressed. I want to look ahead, and take one day at a time.

Mothers who were having memories were then asked to "describe the general or specific memories you have been experiencing during the past month in as much detail as you'd like." After describing each recent memory, mothers rated that memory as being emotionally painful, pleasurable, or neutral. Overall, 79% of these mothers at 6 months and 84% at 18 months described painful memories, but almost as many described pleasurable memories. As Figure 8.1 portrays, most of the mothers having memories reported a combination of pleasurable and painful memories, and did so even more as time passed.

Figure 8.2 lists the specific memories we classified and the percentages of mothers reporting them at each folow-up. The only difference in the manifest content of mothers' memories across the year separating the interviews was that approximately 3 times as many mothers found themselves recalling images of the NICU itself or the apparatus of their child's treatment at 18 months than they had at 6 months.

> Even when my son is grown and he's 6 feet tall, I know I'll look at him sometimes and see him so tiny, hooked up to all those tubes and machines. That's the one picture that will stay in my mind as long as I live.

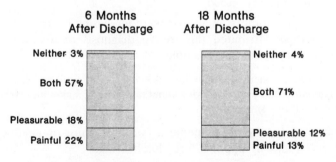

FIGURE 8.1. Percentages of mothers describing pleasurable memories, painful memories, both, or neither.

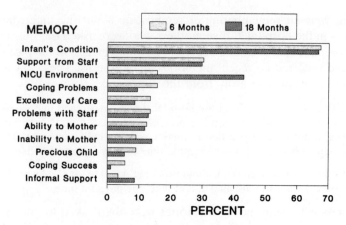

FIGURE 8.2. Percentages of mothers describing specific memories.

The more time that passes, the less I find myself having any memories. But, every time I even go near a hospital, I'll start to have this queasy feeling, and pictures flash in my mind of that unit and all those babies who were fighting for their lives.

The results summarized in Figure 8.2 refer only to the content of mothers' memories, not their frequency or intensity. Most mothers (73%) at 18 months described a steady decline in the frequency of their memories, although some mothers, such as the woman quoted next, found the emotional intensity of their memories undiminished.

My memories are less frequent now, but when I have them, they're just as upsetting. Those memories include the feelings and images of feeling helpless, the sensations of holding such a fragile baby in my arms, the immense frustration I had with some of the doctors, and the suffocating fear that something could go wrong at any second.

For 14% of the mothers, memories were increasing in frequency. Some of these mothers attributed this to the diagnosis of a developmental disability in their child. For example,

My memories are increasing now because he's having more problems with his development. When I start worrying about his future, it makes me start thinking about how all this started.

Others connected the rise in memories with becoming pregnant again or active decision-making about future childbearing.

The more I think about becoming pregnant again, the more memories I start to have of that time. Although he's doing fine now, it was an awful experience that could happen again. It reminds me that I need to take a lot more control over the decisions that are made about my pregnancy.

Painful Memories

Some mothers' distressing memories were quite specific, recapturing powerful emotions and images:

> I still have these flashbacks, like nightmares when you're awake. I see him on the respirator, I hear the doctors telling me that they can't do anything for him, I'm being asked if I'd like him baptized.

> I remember like it was yesterday the day he stopped breathing in my arms. The nurse came over, shook him hard, and he started breathing again.

> Sometimes I'll be driving in the car, and the whole experience will come back to mind. I see myself in the intensive care unit. I see the doctors and nurses bustling about, and I picture myself standing next to the isolette.

> I remember this one nurse who wouldn't let us take him to the family room because she said she was responsible for his whereabouts. . . and another nurse who told us not to watch him choking and gagging when she was inserting a tube in his throat because it made her nervous.

> I remember the fear, that terrifying feeling in the pit of my stomach. I remember all the sights and sounds of that place.

The most common painful memories brought back to mind how sick or close to death the baby had been,

> I remember all those times I called the hospital just to find out if he had survived the night.

> I have memories of how worried I was all the time about whether she was going to make it, whether she was going to live through the day or not.

how hard it had been for them to adjust to this experience,

> The feeling of being by myself without understanding what was happening comes back from time to time. I think this memory will be with me until the day I die.

> I have memories of the scary feeling that everything was completely out of my hands. . . that nothing I could do was going to make any difference.

difficulties in relationships with NICU personnel,

> Most of my memories are still painful, recalling the stress I had dealing with the doctors and the nurses.

> I remember the feeling I got from the doctors and nurses that I didn't belong, that I was just an annoyance, that my baby was just a specimen to them.

and the emptiness they had felt from their inability to be full-time parents,

> The strongest memory I have is this feeling of not being able to care for my baby, this feeling of giving birth to a child who wasn't really yours.

> I remember all the things I wished I could have done to care for him in the hospital, but couldn't, like being able to give him his first bath.

Pleasurable Memories

At the same time, only 22% of the mothers at 6 months and 13% at 18 months were having *only* painful memories of newborn intensive care. Nearly as many mothers reported pleasurable memories as distressing ones, and most described both comforting and upsetting remembrances. Just as some mothers recalled specific distressing events, others described specific events that they were recalling with fondness and satisfaction. Often, these events captured the caring attitudes of the nursing staff:

> I have these memories of one nurse and what she did one day. I came in late one afternoon to learn that they had to shave his head to put an IV in his scalp. Apparently the nurse saw the hair on the floor and put it in an envelope, wrote "my first haircut" on it, and taped it to the side of the isolette. What's nice to remember is that she made a frightening experience into a pleasurable one, just by this small act of kindness.

> I keep remembering this one incident. I came onto the unit and couldn't find him. Then I saw one of the nurses holding him and showing him off to everyone. It made me feel so happy that she loved him so much that she wanted to hold him and play with him.

> I remember like it was yesterday the day she reached three pounds. It was Labor day, and the nurses were so nice to tape a note on the isolette that read "Mommy, be proud of me. I'm three pounds today. Happy Labor Day!"

Some recurring memories of this crisis were always happy ones. These included recollections of support from family, friends, and professionals,

> I find myself remembering how everyone there was so friendly, how they'd go out of their way to answer all my questions. As bad as it was, they made me feel at home, that I belonged there.

the excellent medical care their child had received,

> I have these memories of how well they cared for her, how it saved her life.

> I'm happy when I remember how lucky we were that a place like the unit existed, that there were such competent professionals who cared so much about their work.

and moments of closeness with the child,

> I remember the times when I would look in on her, how she would turn her head when she heard my voice, how she would melt in our arms when we held her, and how, when she was fussy, I would hold her until she'd fall asleep in my arms.

> I remember the first time I touched her. She seemed to know it was me, her mother. I remember the first time I held her, and how happy that made me.

Are Mothers' Memories Mood Congruent?

One factor that might account for differences in the emotional valence of mothers' memories may be their current mood. Blaney (1986) reviewed a wealth of evidence supporting the hypothesis that people's memories of events are "mood congruent," meaning that people who are happy (or sad) are likely to recall happy (or sad) events from their past. Most of the mood congruence studies reviewed by Blaney compare the memories elicited from individuals who differ in depressed mood. In one category of studies, individuals are induced through imagery or hypnotic techniques to feel depressed. In another, people who are clinically depressed or score higher on self-report inventories of depression are compared with nondepressed control individuals. These studies show that when these temporarily or naturally depressed individuals are asked to reminisce about the past, they more frequently recall sad experiences.

Are mothers who were currently more depressed more apt to have unpleasant memories of their child's hospitalization? We addressed this question by inspecting relations between mothers' depressed/elated mood as reported on the Profile of Mood States and the emotional quality of their memories at each time. These relations were not statistically significant, nor were there significant relations between depressed/elated mood and any of the more common specific memories that mothers described as painful or pleasurable. Thus, we have no evidence supporting a "mood congruent" bias in mothers' recall of painful events of the hospitalization.

One reason for this negative finding may be that many mothers were able to refocus their attention on their child's current wellness when they found themselves remembering painful circumstances. In fact, almost half the mothers who recounted memories of how sick or close to death their baby had been volunteered how they sometimes connected these recollections with reminders of their child's current well-being. Blaney (1986) raised the possibility of similar "antidepressive" control mechanisms that attenuate the recall of negative events when one is in a depressed mood. The following quote illustrates how one mother's upsetting memories of her child in the hospital were occasioned by her depressed mood but could be interrupted by reminding herself of her child's good outcome:

> When I'm in a sad mood, I find myself picturing him being so sick, seeing him with all those tubes, and remembering what awful things he had to go through. I'll almost start to cry. *But then, I start to think how well he's doing now and I start feeling happy.*

Are Memories Perceived as Helpful or Harmful?

We also explored how mothers evaluate the benefits and harms of their recurring memories. On the one hand, memories of newborn intensive care could be an unwelcome burden in mothers' efforts to cope with their child's caregiving demands after NICU discharge. Some mothers may wish to put the past behind them and focus their attention on current demands, or even on the current pleasures of caregiving. Others may feel that reminiscences of valued experiences and events associated with their child's stay in the intensive care unit enhance their sense of well-being and help them to contend with current realities.

Only 3% of the mothers at 6 months and 7% of those queried at 18 months thought that it was harmful for them to continue to have memories of newborn intensive care. Thirty-five percent at 6 months and 33% at 18 months thought that it was neither helpful nor harmful. Most at each time believed that their memories were in some way helpful. Those who described their memories as helpful said that they reminded them of the personal gains they had made during that time, their child's special needs, how precious their child is, and helped them to appreciate how much progress their child had made. The following quotes illustrate these perceived benefits:

> I like to remember that time. It helped me to put things into their proper perspective. I faced it, I dealt with it. And because of that, it won't be a heartache for the rest of my life.

> It's good for me to remember how sick she was in the hospital. If she catches a cold, it will be worse for her because of her problems. So I do want to remember her past.

> When I look back on that time, I feel thankful. I think how lucky I am to have her at all.

> Sometimes when I'm feeding him, I'll start to remember how difficult he was to feed in the hospital. Then I'll compare that with how much he eats now, and that makes me feel happy.

The Emotional Significance of Involuntary Memories

Another objective was to identify the environmental cues that evoke mothers' memories and how they respond emotionally to these reminders. Current theory (Horowitz, 1983) and research (Affleck, Tennen et al., 1985; Cella, Perry, Kulchycky, & Goodwin, 1988; Horowitz et al., 1979; Lehman et al., 1987; Silver et al., 1983) emphasize the distressing quality of unbidden memories of stressful events. The possibility that involuntary memories of an aversive event can elicit positive emotions has not been formally studied.

Mothers were asked at both interviews whether, during the past month, "any things or events had triggered involuntary memories of the time when your child was in the hospital." After describing these reminders, they characterized their typical emotional response to each as being emotionally pleasurable, emotionally painful, or emotionally neutral.

As Figure 8.3 indicates, 76% of the mothers described reminders of the hospitalization in the 6th month after discharge, and 81% did so in the 18th

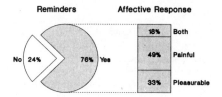

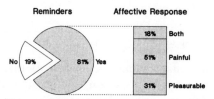

FIGURE 8.3. Percentages of mothers describing pleasurable reminders, painful reminders, or both.

month. The largest proportion of mothers reported only painful reminders at each time, but a substantial number had encountered only pleasurable reminders.

Table 8.1 presents what mothers identified as major reminders of their child's intensive care and the percentage of mothers who described pleasurable, painful, or emotionally neutral responses to these memory cues. In addition to these major categories of reminders, some mothers called attention to evocative stimuli that they associated with the hospitalization. For example,

> Sometimes, when I'm cleaning house a song will play on the radio that was popular then, and it starts to rekindle memories.

> Sometimes the buzzer on the clothes dryer will go off, and it brings back the feeling of being in the unit, with all those monitors sounding off.

> Everytime my eye catches the scars in her arm from the IV, I start to remember what she looked like in the hospital. I remember how much I hated seeing her like that.

Painful Reminders

As current theory (Horowitz, 1983) and previous research (Cella et al., 1988; Lehman et al., 1987; Silver et al., 1983) predict, many mothers

TABLE 8.1. Percentages of mothers reporting specific painful, neutral, and pleasurable reminders of newborn intensive care.

Reminder	Affective response (%)		
	Painful	Neutral	Pleasurable
Media reports on newborn intensive care/premature	38.8	9.7	18.4
babies	(34.7)	(6.5)	(15.2)
Early photographs of infant	8.7	0.0	8.7
	(9.7)	(2.2)	(13.0)
Hearing about or seeing infants with similar history	8.7	3.9	8.7
	(10.8)	(2.2)	(9.8)
Others' comments/questions about child's appearance/	8.7	8.7	18.5
progress	(3.3)	(3.3)	(0.0)
Hearing about or seeing expectant mothers	8.7	3.9	0.0
	(3.3)	(3.3)	(0.0)
Hearing about or seeing healthy babies or deliveries	5.9	2.9	0.0
	(3.3)	(3.3)	(0.0)
Visits to pediatrician	3.9	0.0	6.8
	(7.6)	(4.4)	(4.4)

[a] First number is at 6 mos. Second number (in parens) is at 18 mos.

described painful reminders of their child's hospitalization. One set of memory cues—seeing or hearing about an expectant mother, normal delivery, or healthy newborn—almost always elicited unpleasant emotions among mothers who reported them. We suspect that these events evoked sadness or regret because they set the stage for envious comparisons between their own and other mothers' more successful experience with pregnancy and delivery. One mother described it this way:

> A woman in my office was discussing what it is like to take care of a newborn baby. That got me to remembering what I had missed. I felt an empty space because I'll never know what that is like. I only knew what it was like to come home from the hospital and worry.

Others mentioned how questions and comments about the child started them recalling painful times,

> Every time I have to explain to nosy people why he's so small for his age, it brings back memories of how scared I was waiting for things to get better.

as did learning about the birth of a premature infant to an acquaintance,

> I have heard that two of our neighbors have just had a premature baby. When I think of what they must be going through, it frightens me to recall what I went through.

and visits to the pediatrician,

> Whenever I have to bring my baby to the doctor for a check-up, and I watch him doing the examination, I get very upset because I start to imagine him on the unit, with all those people examining him like he's some guinea pig and not my child.

Pleasurable Reminders

Previous research has not considered the possibility that reminders of a threatening event might also trigger pleasurable emotions. Nonetheless, this was confirmed by many mothers, who described positive emotions at least some of the times they were reminded of their child's hospitalization. Interestingly, many of the same cues that were identified by some mothers as eliciting painful emotions were associated by others with pleasurable feelings. Compare, for example, the comments of these two mothers:

> Stories I see on TV bring it all back to me. I start to see him on the respirator, hear the doctors telling me that they can't do anything for him, and feel how it was to be alone, not understanding what was happening.

> There's quite a bit on the news about preemies these days. But it doesn't haunt me. In fact, I begin to remember fondly how the nurses helped me through it all...how nice it was to be around them.

Some mothers tried to elicit these cherished feelings by doing things to remind themselves of that time.

> When I reminisce about this time, I remember how nice people were to us. I saved all of their cards and take them out from time to time just to remind myself how wonderful it was to be loved and cared about.

> Some nights, I will sit down and look through the photographs that were taken of him in the hospital. This brings back to mind the tremendous changes he went through, from a sick baby who was close to death to the healthy happy baby I have with me now. What a nice feeling that is!

Predicting Mothers' Emotional Response to Reminders

Our next aim was to examine selected predictors of mothers' emotional response to reminders of the newborn intensive care crisis. Horowitz (1983) theorized that the decline of involuntary painful memroies of a traumatic experience depends on "changes in inner models of the self, others, and the world" (p. 130). This general view of the process of coping with stressful events has much in common with Janoff-Bulman and Frieze's (1983) analysis of the reconstruction of the "assumptive world," Taylor's (1983) theory of cognitive adaptation, and Thompson and Janigian's (1988) discussion of the restoration of "life schemes" after victimization. These authors agree that coping with victimization can be assisted by cognitive adaptations that help to restore cherished assumptions. Silver et al. (1983) found a decline in intrusive, upsetting memories among incest victims who had been able to find some meaning in their victimization. Thus, we anticipated that mothers who had perceived greater personal control over their infant's recovery in the hospital, had construed a purpose in crisis, or had described benefits and gains from this experience would later find themselves experiencing less painful (or more pleasurable) emotional responses to reminders of newborn intensive care. Mothers' perceptions of their personal control over their child's recovery and progress in the NICU were elicited by the 11-point rating scale described in chapter 4. In a previous study (Affleck, Tennen et al., 1985), mothers of medically fragile infants described their answers, if any, to the question "Why me? Why was I the one who had a baby who needed to be hospitalized in an intensive care unit?" The five most common responses suggesting the discovery of a purpose in this crisis were presented to mothers in the current study. These statements were: (a) We're better able than most parents to care for a sick baby; (b) This happened so that I could learn something important about myself; (c) God picks parents who can cope with this problem; (d) This challenge is a test of my faith; and (e) God selected me to give special care to this child. Mothers who agreed with any of these statements were classified as having discovered a purpose in the crisis. Finally, mothers who agreed with the statement that "nothing good at all has come out of this experience" were compared with those who disagreed with this statement.

Several investigators (e.g., Affleck, Tennen et al., in press; Chesler & Barbarin, 1984; Lehman et al., 1986) have shown that the ability to obtain appropriate support from family and friends can have pronounced effects on people's adjustment to stressful events. In the case of a health-care problem, the ability to negotiate a satisfying partnership with care providers appears especially critical (Reid, 1984). In Chapter 7, we discussed the role of mothers' social support in their well-being. In Chapter 4, we underscored the benefits of satisfying relationships with health-care professionals on the NICU. Accordingly, we hypothesized that mothers' affective response to reminders of their child's intensive care would depend, in part, on their evaluation of the social support they had obtained during their child's hospitalization and their ability to build an effective partnership with their infant's care providers. At NICU discharge, mothers answered four questions on the Arizona Social Support Scale (Barrera, 1981; see Chapter 7 for a complete description). At NICU discharge, mothers were asked to describe how they felt about their involvement in important decisions that were made about their child's care and treatment (see Chapter 4.) From these responses, they were classified into two groups: those who had encountered no problems in this area and those who reported difficulties in attaining control over decision-making, being adequately informed about treatments before they were carried out, or both.

A person's emotional state during a stressful event is represented in his long-term memory of the crisis (Horowitz, 1983). Thus, mothers' mood during their child's hospitalization could also influence how they feel when they are reminded later of this time. Further, the predictive significance of cognitive adaptations, social support, and relationships with care providers may be due to their effects on mothers' general emotional well-being before NICU discharge. Therefore, mothers' scores on the Profile of Mood States at NICU discharge were also incorporated in the predictive analyses. Along with these predictive questions, we examined whether mothers' longer term emotional response to reminders of newborn intensive care might be influenced by the child's developmental outcome, as Philipp (1983) hypothesized.

Predicting Painful Reminders

The only variable predicting the occurrence of painful reminders at 6 months was the description of problems with NICU staff. After controlling for background characteristics, mothers' problems with NICU staff were still a factor in their experience of painful reminders at 6 months. In this multiple regression equation, mothers of first-born children and mothers of infants with more severe medical problems were also more likely to identify painful reminders at 6 months. The only variable predicting painful reminders at 18 months was the conclusion that there were no benefits or gains ensuing from the hospitalization. This association remained significant even when the background variables and the infant's developmental outcome at 18 months were taken into account.

Predicting Pleasurable Reminders

Four variables measured before discharge predicted pleasurable reminders at 6 months: positive mood, support satisfaction, no problems reported with NICU staff, and finding a purpose in the crisis. When background variables and these four predictors were considered together in a regression analysis, the ability to find a purpose alone remained a significant predictor of pleasurable reminders. The only variable predicting (the absence of) pleasurable reminders at 18 months, once again, was having found no benefits or gains from the experience. Additionally, mothers of children who were not diagnosed as developmentally disabled were more likely to be responding pleasurably to reminders of the hospitalization. When these two correlates of pleasurable reminders were considered along with background variables in a regression analysis, the inability to find benefits or gains was still a factor in the absence of positive responses to reminders.

Intrusive Thoughts and Avoidance of Reminders

So far, our analysis of mothers' remembrances has focused on the occurrence of pleasurable and painful memories and difference in emotional responses to reminders. Another important question concerns the *frequency* with which mothers experienced intrusive thoughts and feelings about the hospitalization and were making efforts to avoid these reminders. An associated question is whether these responses are connected with mothers' psychological well-being and can be predicted by their efforts to cope with their child's hospitalization.

Six and eighteen months after discharge, mothers completed the Impact of Event Scale (Horowitz et al., 1979). This 15-item questionnaire supplies scores for the frequency during the past week of *intrusion* and *avoidance* responses to stressful events. Intrusion items refer to "unbidden thoughts and images, troubled dreams, strong pangs or waves of feelings, and repetitive behavior" and avoidance items reflect "denial of the meanings and consequences of the event, blunted sensations, behavioral inhibition, and awareness of emotional numbness" (Horowitz et al., 1979, p. 210). Examples of intrusion items are "I thought about it when I didn't mean to," "Pictures about it popped into my mind," and "Any reminder brought back feelings about it." Illustrative avoidance items are "I stayed away from reminders of it," "I tried not to think about it," "I tried to remove it from memory."

At each follow-up, intrusion and avoidance scores were significantly correlated, a pattern consistent with Horowitz's (1983) formulation of an oscillating stress response pattern wherein intrusive thoughts are followed by avoidance, which in turn may prompt more intrusive thoughts. Also, both intrusion scores and avoidance scores were correlated over time, indicating that the ordering of mothers on these variables was moderately stable in the year between the assessments. Although mothers as a group experienced fewer intrusive thoughts at 18 months than they had a year previously, their avoidance scores as a group remained about the same during that year.

Relations of Intrusion/Avoidance with Well-Being

Table 8.2 shows that intrusion and avoidance scores related significantly to concurrent measures of mothers' well-being and adaptation. Mothers who were having more intrusive thoughts at 6 months were more depressed and experienced more negative mood states. Similarly, at 18 months their intrusive thoughts correlated with negative mood and global distress. The same was true for relations between avoidance and emotional well-being at each time. In addition, mothers who at 6 months were more avoidant of reminders felt less competent as caregivers.

The availability of repeated reliable measurements of mood, intrusion, and avoidance makes a cross-lagged panel analysis feasible (Kenny, 1975). This procedure, which can determine whether change in one variable predicts change in another, considers together the temporal stabilities of each variable, the synchronous correlations between the two variables, and the cross-time correlations of the variables. Using this technique, we inspected the cross-correlations involving mood and intrusion and then

TABLE 8.2. Correlates of mothers' intrusive thoughts and avoidance of reminders.

Variable	Intrusion		Avoidance	
	6 mos.	18 mos.	6 mos.	18 mos.
Mothers' age	−.16	−.01	−.22*	−.08
Mothers' education	−.13	−.04	−.18	−.05
First-born child	.03	.03	.13	.00
Medical severity	.02	.03	−.09	.07
Mood at discharge	−.13	−.24*	−.30**	−.21*
At 6 months				
Mood	−.23*	−.13	−.28**	−.33**
Depression	.23*	.25*	.30**	.41**
Perceived attachment	−.02	−.08	−.10	−.30**
Sense of competence	−.13	.00	−.23*	−.18
Responsiveness	−.08	−.19	−.10	−.37**
At 18 months				
Mood	−.13	−.22*	−.14	−.34**
Global distress	.13	−.36**	.21*	.42**
Home environment	−.11	.13	−.14	−.08
Developmental status	−.16	−.02	−.18	−.11

* $p < .05$.
** $p < .01$.

involving mood and avoidance. The mood-intrusion analysis yielded no significant results: mood and intrusion were related at each time, but neither predicted the other over time. But, there was support for the hypothesis that mood disturbance leads to greater avoidance, rather than the reverse. The difference between the two cross-correlations presented in Figure 8.4 was statistically significant even when the synchronous relations and stabilities of the variables were taken into account.

Coping Strategies as Predictors of Intrusion/Avoidance

Finally, we examined whether mothers' strategies of coping with newborn intensive care (see Chapter 6) predicted their intrusive thoughts and avoidant responses. We wondered, for example, whether mothers who attempted to escape the problem before discharge might continue to

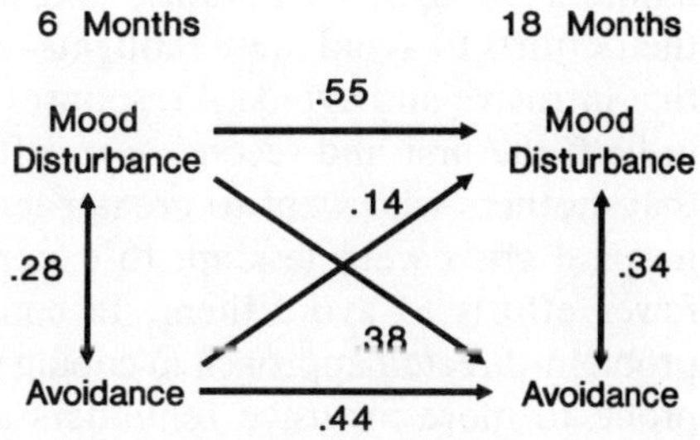

FIGURE 8.4. Cross-lagged panel analysis of mothers' mood disturbance and avoidance of the intensive care crisis.

exhibit avoidant responses months later. Indeed, this was the case at both 6 and 18 months after discharge. Whereas no other coping strategy predicted avoidance, two coping strategies predicted intrusion. Mothers who had minimized the situation reported less intrusion at each follow-up assessment, and mothers who had taken more instrumental actions experienced more intrusion at 18 months.

To determine whether these relations might be accounted for by background variables and mothers' mood at hospital discharge, hierarchical regression models were evaluated. Mothers who minimized still reported less intrusion at 6 and 18 months, and mothers who had done more instrumental action coping still reported more intrusion at 18 months. However, the predictive relation between escapist coping and avoidance did not hold up when these factors were taken into account. This was because mothers who were more emotionally distressed at discharge had used more escapist coping and were also prone to more avoidance later on.

A related question is whether coping strategies might predict patterns of increasing or decreasing intrusion and avoidance across the first two years after discharge. The only coping strategy that met this condition was taking instrumental actions. Controlling for background variables, mothers' mood at discharge, and the level of intrusion reported at 6 months, mothers who used this strategy to a greater extent continued to report more intrusion at 18 months. The inference that can be drawn from this procedure is that mothers who had done more instrumental action coping experienced increasingly more intrusive thoughts of their child's hospitalization as time passed.

The findings reported in this chapter break new ground on the psychological meaning and adaptational significance of mothers' recurring memories of their child's hospitalizaton on a NICU. We revealed the complexity of mothers' memories of this stressful event. Most found themselves remembering both painful and pleasurable aspects of the hospital stay. Many memories—both happy and sad—were evoked involuntarily by events or environmental cues. As we had predicted, mothers' ability to find meaning in this crisis and inability to forge a satisfying relationship with their infant's health-care providers played a part in how they felt when they were reminded of that time. Finally, we examined the intrusiveness of mothers' thoughts, emotions, and memories of the hospitalization and their efforts to avoid these thoughts, emotions, and reminders. We showed that intrusive and avoidant responses accompanied signs of maladaptation in both the first and second years after discharge. We also demonstrated that mothers who went to greater lengths to minimize the severity of the hospital crisis were less apt to experience intrusive memories and made fewer efforts to avoid them. In contrast, those who had taken a more problem-directed approach in coping with their child's hospitalization were prone to more intrusive reminders and experienced increasing levels of intrusion over a year's time.

This chapter brings to a close our analysis of the nature, determinants, and consequences of mothers' cognitive adaptations, appraisals of social support, and coping strategies. Before summarizing and discussing our key findings, we examine the crisis of newborn intensive care from one last perspective—the difference and similarities between mothers and fathers and between husbands and wives.

9
Mothers, Fathers, and Couples

The crisis of newborn intensive care is usually faced by a mother, a father, and a couple. This was true in 90% of the families in our study. Although researchers have found a correspondence between the quality of a mother's relationship with her premature infant and the quality of her relationship with her husband (e.g., Herzog, 1979), they have not examined this association in fathers of preterm infants. Little is known as well about differences between mothers' and fathers' adaptations and adjustment; concordances of distress, appraisals, and coping strategies within couples; the effect of one partner's coping strategies on the other partner's well-being; the implications of coping similarities and differences for the marital relationship; or the perceived impact of this crisis on the marital relationship. This chapter addresses these questions in analyses of data gathered at NICU discharge and 18 months later from our subgroup of 50 married mothers and their husbands.

Distress and Well-Being

Several researchers have shown that fathers are less upset than mothers by the hospitalization of a medically fragile newborn (Benfield, Leib, & Reuter, 1979; Jeffcoate et al., 1979; Philipp, 1976; Trause & Kramer, 1983). But this finding can be questioned because of flaws in these researchers' sampling methods and statistical analyses. Only some participants in these studies were married to other participants. More important, the marital relationship was not usually taken into account in statistical analyses.

For this and other comparisons reported in this chapter, we address two questions. One is whether mothers as a group differ from fathers as a group. Statistical analyses of this type of comparison take account the fact that half the informants were married to the other half, that is, that responses come from "matched pairs." The other type of comparison we report is within couples. Regardless of any differences that might exist between mothers and fathers, how much does a wife's response correspond with her husband's?

There was no relation between husbands and wives in their mood at NICU discharge or in their mood and global distress at 18 months. This indicates that a parent's well-being does not depend on his spouse's well-being across the phases of this threatening event. At the same time, mothers reported more overall mood disturbance at NICU discharge than did fathers. This finding is consistent with research showing that stressful events in general are more upsetting to women than to men (Bolger, DeLongis, Kessler, & Schilling, 1989; Solomon & Rothblum, 1986; Wethington, McLeod, & Kessler, 1987). It suggests that fathers are less uspet than mothers by the hospitalization of a newborn on an intensive care unit. To some extent, as we discuss more fully below, this may be due to fathers' ability to find effective coping strategies for alleviating distress. Mothers' greater distress could also stem from their more negative assessment of the infant's current and future problems. Levy-Shiff, Sharir, and Mogilner (1989) showed that mothers perceived their hospitalized premature infant to be more difficult than did fathers. And more mothers than fathers in the current study, as we report in the next section, were concerned with future problems of health and development.

Other interpretations of this finding are plausible. First, gender differences in early mood may be due, in part, to some mothers' recovery from obstetric surgery or to postpartum mood disorder and thus may have little to do with their reaction to the hospitalization itself. Second, fathers may simply be more reluctant to admit disturbing responses in a mood checklist. This explanation is questioned by the similar findings reported by other investigators who have used different methods of assessing mothers' and fathers' emotional adaptation to the birth of a premature infant (Benfield et al., 1976; Jeffcoate et al., 1979; Trause & Kramer, 1983) and to the loss of a baby in the perinatal period (Rowe, Clyman, Green, Mikkelsen, Haight, & Ataide, 1978; Walwork & Ellison, 1985). A third interpretation is the possibility that more fathers than mothers try to minimize their outward emotional response to this crisis. In fact, this distinction was captured in the comments of the many mothers who described their husband's coping style as "keeping his feelings in"; interestingly, no husband characterized his wife's coping in this way. This explanation is strengthened by evidence that negative emotions are more aversive to men than to women (Gottman & Levenson, 1988). Hence, men may try harder to bring their emotions into equilibrium.

This difference in mood between mothers and fathers persisted to 18 months after discharge. Our global distress index at 18 months, however, did not differentiate mothers from fathers. On SCL-90R subscales that tap emotional reactions, that is, depression, anxiety, and hostility subscales, mothers scored higher, consistent with the mood scale findings. But on other subscales, including one that captures a different type of response to distress—somatization—fathers were very much like mothers. The somatization items cover physical symptoms involving the cardiovascular, gastrointestinal, and respiratory systems. Therefore, although mothers appear more distraught, they do not exhibit other stress reactions to a greater extent. This strengthens our inference that fathers may have other ways of manifesting distress than are exhibited by emotional disequilibrium. One mother commented on this difference in terms of her and her husband's way of handling the stress of this event:

> I cried a lot and talked a lot about the problem and how I was feeling upset. He didn't cry and he wouldn't talk about his feelings. But at times he would start to drink too much and he would need to take medication to control his "nerves."

Appraisals of Control, Outcome, and Meaning

Comparisons of mothers' and fathers' appraisals of control over the child's outcome, their expectations of their child's future health and development, and their ability to find meaning in this crisis have not been the subject of prior research. To review our method, each parent rated on a scale of 0 = "no control" to 10 = "extreme amount of control" the extent to which the infant's recovery and progress in the NICU depended on things that he or she had done. Then, each described the specific activities that afforded him or her a sense of control over the infant's recovery. Next, each parent estimated the probability (on a scale of 0–100%) that the infant's future health and development "would be normal in all respects." Parents were then asked to described what, if any, problems of health and development they were even slightly concerned might eventuate.

Mothers reported more personal control over their infant's recovery than did fathers. Categories of personal control activities offered by mothers and fathers included visiting the unit frequently, providing social stimulation, providing nonsocial stimulation, carrying out caregiving tasks, monitoring treatment procedures, and praying. McNemar tests showed that mothers were significantly more likely than fathers to mention social stimulation as an activity that gave them a sense of control over their infant's recovery. This parellels findings reported by Levy-Shiff et al. (1989) that mothers actually spend more time than fathers talking to their premature newborns in the hospital. A moderately high correlation obtained between spouses' perceptions of control suggests that some couples may have been able to share in a joint sense of efficacy. Interestingly, many used the subject "we" instead of "I" in describing what they did to gain control.

Unlike gender differences in control appraisals, mothers and fathers did not differ in their general expectations of a normal outcome. At the same time, a wife's expectation did correspond with her husband's. Parent's reported concerns about their child's future development and health included the possibilities of mental retardation, sensory disabilities, motor

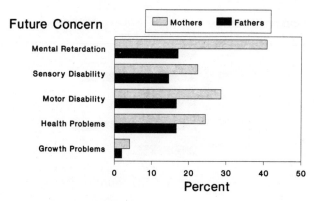

FIGURE 9.1. Percentages of mothers and fathers expressing concerns about their infant's future health and development.

disabilities, health problems, and growth problems. Figure 9.1 presents the comparisons between mothers' and fathers' future concerns. McNemar tests showed that significantly more mothers than fathers mentioned at least a slight concern with the possibility that their child would be mentally retarded. Mothers also expressed significantly more concerns about their infant's future health and development than did fathers.

Mothers and fathers were also compared on their agreement with two statements reflecting the inability to find meaning in this event: (1) Nothing good has come from this experience, and (2) There is no reason or purpose why this happened. Marital partners were not concordant for their agreement with these statements, and mothers or fathers as a group did not differ in their endorsement of these beliefs.

Coping Strategies

Differences between mothers and fathers and concordances within couples in the use of strategies of coping with newborn intensive care have also been ignored in previous research. Mothers' and fathers' coping strategies during their infant's hospitalization were measured by the WOCC (see Chapter 6). Figure 9.2 portrays the absolute and relative (proportion of overall coping) scores for mothers and fathers on the five coping strategies measured by this questionnaire. Significant differences in the distribution of coping strategies were evident. Women used more escapist coping than men, both in absolute and relative terms. They also expended greater effort to mobilize support. This finding is consistent with research showing that women seek more support than men in coping with adversity (Fleishman, 1984; Heppner, Reeder, & Larson, 1983; Stanton et al., 1990; Stone & Neale, 1984). At the same time, support mobilization did not occupy a greater relative role in mothers' overall coping efforts. The

120   9. Mothers, Fathers, and Couples

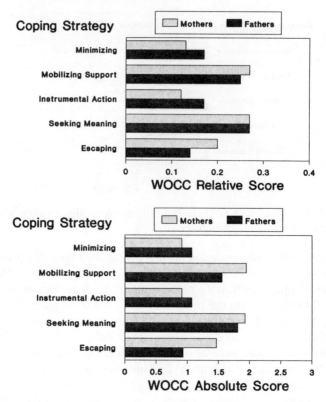

FIGURE 9.2. Mean absolute and relative scores on the Ways of Coping Checklist (WOCC) for mothers and fathers.

coping strategies of fathers included greater relative, but no absolute, use of minimization and instrumental actions.

There were also relations within couples in the use of coping strategies. When one spouse scored higher in the relative use of minimization, seeking meaning or support mobilization, the other tended to score higher on these coping strategies as well. Husbands' absolute levels of escapist coping and seeking meaning also correlated with their wives'.

Coping Strategies and Well-Being

In Chapter 6, where we examined concurrent relations between relative coping strategies and mood in the total sample of mothers, two significant findings were reported. Mothers who had done more minimizing expressed more positive mood, and those who had done more escaping expressed more negative mood. For the subgroup of married mothers incorporated in this analysis, escaping, but not minimizing, was a correlate of negative mood ($r = -.39, p < .01$). For their husbands, escaping was also correlated with negative mood ($r = -.42, p < .01$), minimizing was correlated with positive mood ($r = .36, p < .05$), and taking instrumental action was also correlated with positive mood ($r = .39, p < .01$). There was one difference between mothers and fathers in this pattern of correlations: among fathers, the association between taking instrumental action and positive mood was significantly greater than the relation between these variables for mothers. There were no significant associations between a parent's coping strategies and the mood reported by his or her partner. Whereas mothers' and fathers' coping strategies were implicated in their own emotional well-being at NICU discharge, they were not a factor in their spouse's well-being.

The previously reported association between mothers' inclination to seek meaning in the crisis and less global distress 18 months later was echoed in our smaller sample of married mothers ($r = -.32, p < .05$). Although the same was not true for their husbands, the difference in the correlations for mothers and fathers was negligible. Fathers whose coping was characterized by greater minimization were less globally distressed at 18 months ($r = -.38, p < .01$), but again, the correlation for fathers did not differ from that for mothers. Paralleling our findings for mood reports at NICU discharge, no relation was found between one parent's coping strategies and the marital partner's well-being at 18 months.

Appraisals of Coping Differences

The findings reported thus far document key differences between mothers and fathers and between husbands and wives in their distress, appraisal, and coping strategies. In this section, we examine how marital partners themselves assess the meaning and significance of these differences. When asked to describe "similarities and differences in the ways in which you and your spouse have been coping with your child's hospitalization on the newborn intensive care unit," approximately 75% of both mothers and fathers reported coping differences. Before discussing parents' evaluations of these differences, we wish to emphasize through the following remarks how important it was for some spouses to feel that they were approaching this experience in similar ways.

> We've been together on everything, almost like we were one person. We came up with a routine together and we followed it to the letter. We actually spent more time together than we ever had since we got married. My wife and I found new ways to comfort each other, and we both looked for something positive about this.

> We turned to each other for support, we held onto each other, and we looked to God. That made our relationship stronger than it has ever been.

Echoing what we surmised in our discussion of differences in mothers' and fathers' mood reports, the most commonly reported difference, noted by both men and women, was wives' tendency to express their emotional distress and husbands' inclination to dampen their outward expression of distress:

> He held things in, but not me. I knew he was worried and upset, but he wouldn't come out and say it.

> My wife was more tearful and sad. I couldn't always understand what was upsetting her. I thought it was important for me to keep things under control.

Parents were asked further to comment on the significance of any coping differences for their own well-being, their spouse's well-being, and the marital relationship. One reason why we did not find any relation between one partner's coping strategies and the other partner's adaptation may be that some saw divergent coping methods as a threat whereas others viewed them as an advantage. Compare, for example, the following unfavorable interpretations of coping differences:

> I would cry and he would yell at the dog. He kept busy at work and I was there with the problem all of the time. This put quite a strain on our relationship. I'd wonder why he didn't react like I did. Didn't he love him too?

> He's been withdrawing from me more and more. I've been pouring out my feelings and he hasn't been showing his at all. This has placed a great strain on our relationship. We're communicating less and less.

> He seemed to always expect the worst and became very nervous about things. I would try to take things in stride and look on the bright side. When I did try to let my emotions out, he couldn't deal with this. These days, we don't communicate as much as we used to. We're not as close as we were before this happened.

> My wife seemed a glutton for punishment. She felt she had to be at the hospital all the time to share in our baby's suffering. She couldn't understand the importance of having a life outside of all of this. I visited the hospital a lot too, but I was trying to deal only with the problems as they arose, waiting to cross the bridges when we came to them. She would say things like "Maybe you don't understand how bad things are, because if you did, you'd be as upset as I am." I was just as upset, but I didn't show it. I was trying to keep the rest of my life in balance. It would have been ridiculous for me to feel what she was feeling. If I had been, I wouldn't have been any good to her at all. I can't understand why she didn't appreciate this. It's very frustrating for me.

with these positive evaluations of similar differences:

> My husband and I coped very differently. I made myself go to the hospital every day, but he would stay away. Once I realized how discouraged he would get by not seeing much progress, it didn't bother me. Actually I came to understand him better, and that brought us closer together.

> I cried more and talked more about it. I think he was trying to keep things in perspective for me. We both realized that what the other person was feeling was okay, even though we had different ways of coping with this problem.

Sometimes, these differences were seen as a mixed blessing:

> He kept things in, I let them out. That has left its scars on our relationship, but at least we're now more aware of how each of us copes with a difficult situation.

Taken a step further, the possibility of mutually helpful, reciprocal coping strategies was suggested by several parents' comparisons of their own and their spouses' coping methods:

> His approach was more objective and logical. He wanted to take things as they came. My approach was more emotional and refusing to think about the possibility of bad things. But I really needed his perspective on things at times.

> I would try to deal with the worst, to dig for the truth. He was always more optimistic and positive. But sometimes that would really help me when I was down.

> She took it a lot harder. She would get down on herself, blame herself. I didn't take it as hard, and tried to keep things in balance. Maybe we were put together so we could deal with problems like this through our differences.

Appraisals of Social Support

Another theme emerging from parents' descriptions of coping differences is that fathers more than mothers seemed to focus their attention on helping their spouse cope with this crisis. As one husband stated,

> My wife is more emotional about things. She was more concerned than I was about our baby's hurting and pain. I'd focus on trying to help her cope by sitting back, listening to her, and then trying to help her become more rational about things.

Some mothers, such as the following woman, also recognized this difference and commented further on their husband's inability to find the support they were obtaining from others:

> I know my husband has spent a lot of time and energy trying to get me through this. He's been very supportive and sensitive to my feelings. But sometimes I worry about how little attention he's been getting from everyone. Sometimes it seems like I've been the center of everyone's concern, and no one, including me, has given enough to him.

This possibility has also raised in studies of couples' coping with the death of a child in the perinatal period (DeFrain, 1986).

This apparent "imbalance" in mutual support did not appear to have had an adverse effect on fathers' evaluations of the social support they had obtained when their child was hospitalized. Fathers were not less satisfied with the support they received from their wives than mothers were with they support they received from their husbands. Despite the fact that some fathers noted a tendency of NICU nurses and physicians to pay more attention to their wife's needs than to their own, their satisfaction with the support they received from nurses and physicians did not differ from mothers' evaluations of these support providers. Moreover, fathers were *more* satisfied than mothers with the overall support they secured during this time. One reason may be that they also reported a lower need for support, which, as we have shown earlier, is a key factor in people's assessments of their social networks. Finally, fathers' mood at NICU discharge was not related to their support satisfaction although it was for mothers. The support-mood relation was also significantly greater for mothers than for fathers. Thus, even fathers who were displeased with their support may not have responded negatively to this appraisal, as did their wives.

Perceived Impact on the Marital Relationship

In Chapter 3, we discussed how many mothers described improvements in the marital relationship as one of the unexpected benefits of this crisis. Macey, Harmon, and Easterbrooks (1987) reported that half of their sample of mothers of premature infants, 1 year after the delivery, described their marriages as closer than they were before the birth. Here, we explore this question in more detail. For this analysis, we drew on each parent's agreement with two statements presented to them at NICU discharge: (1) My baby's hospitalization has brought my spouse and me closer together, and (2) My baby's hospitalization has caused problems in my relationship with my spouse. Ratings of agreement were made on five-point scales. Approximately 70% of both husbands and wives thought that the marital relationship had been moderately or strongly improved, and there was no difference in their agreement with this statement. And when a wife believed this to be true, her husband tended to believe it as well. However, fathers were more likely than mothers to believe that this crisis harmed the marital relationship, and there was not agreement within couples about the extent to which the marriage had been disrupted. For both mothers and fathers, appraisals of marital harm and marital benefit were inversely and highly correlated. Thus, a composite variable reflecting an overall assessment of the impact of the crisis on the marital relationship was constructed for each parent, with higher scores representing a more positive appraisal.

Mothers' and fathers' appraisals of marital impact were not affected by age, education, or parity. Fathers, but not mothers, of the sicker infants were more apt to describe the relationship as being harmed. The marital impact appraisal did not correlate with mood reports at NICU discharge for either husbands or wives. But fathers who described the relationship as more improved reported more positive mood 18 months later ($r = .45$, $p < .05$), and mothers citing improvements reported less global distress at 18 months ($r = -.39, p < .05$). These associations remained significant even when parents' mood at discharge and the severity of the infant's condition were controlled statistically.

Mothers' appraisals of marital impact also predicted children's outcomes at 18 months. Wives who claimed that the relationship was improved by the intensive care crisis had children who enjoyed better outcomes ($r = .39$, $p < .01$). Fathers' perceptions of marital impact did not predict children's outcomes. The difference between the predictive associations for mothers and fathers was statistically significant.

This chapter ends our analysis of separate themes in the process of parents' adaptation to the birth, hospitalization, and home care of medically fragile infants. In the final chapter, we review what we have learned from this study, report summary analyses of the predictors of mothers' longer term adaptation and children's development, and draw implications from this research for helping professionals.

10
Summary and Discussion

Chapters 3 through 9 each address a separate theme in parents' adaptation to newborn intensive care and its aftermath. In this concluding chaper we summarize and discuss the key findings, their broader implications for helping professionals, and additional information about the efficacy of supportive interventions for parents. Before doing so, we present integrative analyses involving the prediction of mothers' longer term well-being, the quality of home environments, and children's developmental outcomes.

Integrative Analyses

Throughout this book we identified many factors that predict a mother's longer term emotional distress, the quality of the support she provides for her child's development, and her child's developmental outcome itself. Now we consider these predictors together to determine their overall and unique contributions to these outcomes. The technique we use, path analysis (Kerlinger & Pedhazur, 1973), allowed us to examine whether predictors at NICU discharge forecast these outcomes directly or are medicated by other predictors measured 6 months after discharge.

Mothers' Global Distress

Thirteen variables were identified as significant predictors of mothers' global distress on the SCL-90R 18 months after discharge. Mothers who became more distressed had before discharge reported less positive mood, expressed less satisfaction with social support, failed to find benefits in the crisis, blamed others for their child's medical problems to a greater extent, were less optimistic about their child's prospects for normal health and development, expected greater control over their child's health and development, engaged in fewer efforts to seek meaning, and engaged in more instrumental action coping. At 6 months, the subsequently more

126

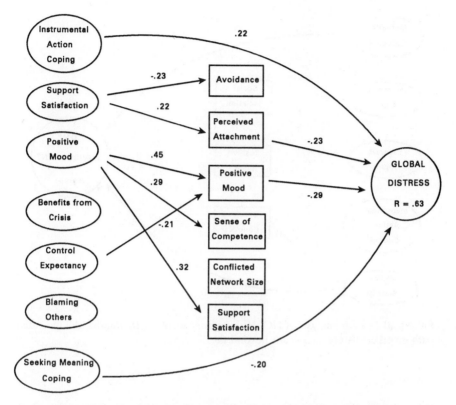

FIGURE 10.1. Path analysis of mothers' SCL-90R Global Severity Index scores at 18 months. All indicated path co-efficients are significant beyond the .05 level.

distressed mothers reported less positive mood, felt less attached to their child, perceived themselves as less competent caregivers, rated their support network as less helpful, reported conflicts over the child with more individuals, and exhibited more avoidant responses to reminders of their child's hospitalization.

Figure 10.1 depicts the predictive relationships between these variables and mothers' global distress, indicating the statistically significant direct and indirect path co-efficients. When all variables in the predictive model were considered, their multiple correlation with distress was .63 ($p < .01$). When the unique role of each variable was considered, that is, controlling for all other predictors, four factors were independent predictors of distress: less positive mood at 6 months, less attachment at 6 months, less reliance on seeking meaning as a coping strategy before discharge, and greater reliance on instrumental actions as a predischarge coping strategy.

As Figure 10.1 shows, three additional variables measured before discharge played an indirect predictive role in mothers' distress owing to

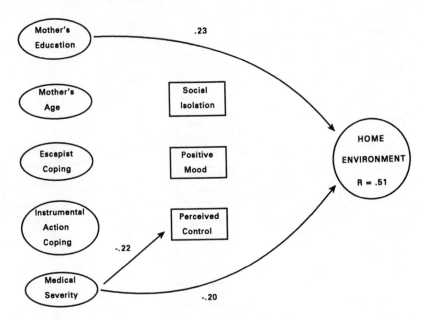

FIGURE 10.2. Path analysis of HOME Inventory scores at 18 months. All indicated path co-efficients are significant beyond the .05 level.

their associations with the two unique predictors at 6 months. Not surprisingly, mothers' mood at discharge played an indirect role because of its prediction of mood at 6 months. But mothers' 6 month mood was also a function of their earlier control expectancies, with those anticipating greater control at discharge reporting more mood disturbance 6 months later. Finally, mothers' support satisfaction before discharge played an indirect role in their subsequent distress because of its association with perceived attachment at 6 months.

Quality of Home Environments

The eight predictors of HOME Inventory scores are presented in the path diagram depicted in Figure 10.2. To summarize, more optimal home environments were found for mothers who were more educated, older, and whose infants' condition was less severe; for mothers who had coped with newborn intensive care by taking greater instrumental actions and making fewer efforts to escape from the problem; and for mothers who reported less social isolation, more positive mood, and greater control over their child's eating and sleeping behavior 6 months after discharge. The multiple correlation between these predictors and HOME scores was .51 ($p < .01$). Two of the variables were unique predictors: medical severity and mothers'

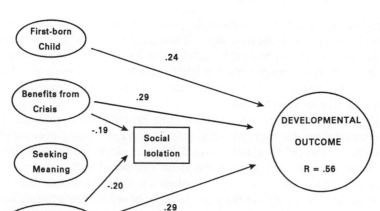

FIGURE 10.3. Path analysis of children's developmental quotients at 18 months. All indicated path co-efficients are significant beyond the .05 level.

education. Thus, it appears that processes related to coping, support, and appraisal were overridden by background variables that predicted home environments.

Children's Development

Finally, the five variables that predicted childrens' developmental outcome are listed in Figure 10.3. Superior developmental outcomes were exhibited by children who were first-born and whose mothers at discharge had construed benefits from the crisis, sought meaning as a coping strategy, and offered more optimistic predictions about the child's development and at 6 months described themselves as more socially isolated. The multiple correlation of these five variables with children's developmental status was .56 ($p < .01$). In addition to parity, two variables played unique predictive roles: construing benefits and holding optimistic outcome expectancies.

Review and Discussion

In Chapters 3 and 4, we explored how parents are able to restore a sense of meaning and mastery in the face of the profound challenges to their "assumptive world" delineated in Chapter 1. We began by documenting numerous ways in which mothers of medically fragile infants pursue the meaning of their child's hazardous delivery, intensive care, and any problems encountered during the transition home. Most were able to reappraise this threatening experience in ways that made a potentially senseless occurrence a meaningful one, or at least a less aversive experience than it might have been. Their capacity to find a purpose in the crisis, their ability to construe benefits and gains from their misfortune, and their proclivity to compare their plight to less desirable alternatives helped them to mitigate a sense of victimization and its accompanying stigmatization and threats to self-esteem.

The ability to find benefits figured most prominently in mothers' long-term adaptation. Mothers who had failed to find something positive about this situation were, 18 months after discharge, more emotionally distressed. This was the case even when their emotional well-being at NICU discharge and the severity of their infant's medical problems were taken into account. Not only did the perception of benefits have a lasting impact on mothers' emotions, but it also predicted how their children would develop in the 2 years after discharge. And as our integrative analyses revealed, the link between perceiving benefits and positive outcomes for the child was a direct one, unmediated by any variables examined at 6 months. Finally, we raised the possibility that some appraised benefits, notably the belief that close relationships were strengthened, signal influential differences in mothers' ability to obtain social support. This appeared to be true in the case of perceived improvements in the marital relationship.

Our findings on mothers' search for mastery over the crisis of newborn intensive care are complex and capture the many nuances in the literature on the advantages and disadvantages of perceived control. Several key distinctions, summarized below, are warranted by our analysis: (a) differences in perceived control over different outcomes; (b) differences among retrospective control appraisals, control expectancies, and outcome expectancies; and (c) variations in the need for control over childrens' medical care in the hospital.

The first distinction supported by our findings is that mothers' retrospective control perceptions are not generalized to all outcomes observed in child. Rather, mothers appear to distinguish their influence over their child's mental development, motor development, and health from their ability to affect their child's sleeping patterns and eating habits. This appears a realistic distinction, reflecting differences between outcomes that are arguably more or less controllable. Yet, it was mothers' perceived control over what might be presumed to be the less controllable outcomes—eating and sleeping—that made the difference in their longer-term well-being and interactions with their child. The reasons for this finding are unclear. Perhaps these mothers were able to find inventive ways of influencing these outcomes. Perhaps those mothers who took personal responsibility for these outcomes had children who ate and slept better. If neither were the case, the illusion of control itself may have been adaptive.

Our results also underscore the distinction of retrospective control appraisals from control expectancies. It is apparent that mothers who could perceive a link between their own activities and their child's current condition in the hospital or after discharge were aided by this perception. This was evidenced in the statistical findings and in mothers' comments during the interview. At the same time, mothers who anticipated that their child's future outcomes would depend on their own actions appeared to encounter greater distress into the second year after discharge. Both our results and the findings of other researchers suggest that expecting control can threaten well-being when attempts to achieve that control come at great personal cost or when departures from the expected outcome are encountered. The fact that mothers who anticipated greater control were not necessarily those who had perceived more control once the outcome was known adds further weight to the distinction between these two appraisals. Many mothers who did not place great emphasis on their ability to affect their child's outcome were, nonetheless, able to look back and connect the outcome to their own behavior.

Mothers who believed that their child's development would depend to a greater extent on their own interventions were not necessarily more confident that the hoped for outcome would be achieved. But expecting a good outcome itself may have had beneficial consequences. Mothers who were more optimistic about their child's future seemed comforted in lasting ways. More important, their child'a actual development may have been enhanced by their positive expectancies, as was indicated in the integrative analysis by the direct path between outcome expectancies and actual outcomes. Perhaps, we speculated, these mothers were better able to normalize their child's care and were spared the urge to overprotect a child perceived as vulnerable and fragile.

Of course, mothers expecting a good outcome were usually correct. This was true in this sample of infants across the 18 months in which they were followed, and would be the case for newborn intensive care graduates in general. Although this fact may account in part for our findings, we also found that mothers who had held positive expectancies and whose children became developmentally disabled experienced no greater distress than those who had held less positive expectations. Thus, the confirmation of the expectancy is not a critical factor in monthers' long-term adaptation.

The last distinction supported by our findings concerns mothers' differing need for control over their child's medical care in the hospital. One group of mothers was able to achieve a satisfying level of participation in their child's care. Presumably, these mothers' need for control was met by their ability to form a partnership with their child's doctors and nurses. They were able to achieve a sense of "participatory control" over their child's care. A second group of mothers felt little need to participate in teir child's treatment. They tended to relinquish their control freely to their child's health-care providers, and were perhaps able to compensate for this loss of personal control by gaining a sense of "vicarious control." The last group of mothers, whose need for control in this situation seemed quite pronounced, was upset by their inability to acquire the control they desired. They expressed severe criticisms of the staff's refusal to involve them in medical decisions or even to inform them of decisions before they were carried out. Unable to take direct personal control over their child's care, they were unable to acquire a sense of participatory control and were unwilling to pursue the benefits of vicarious control.

In Chapter 5, we continued our analysis of the search for meaning and mastery by considering the implications of mothers' ability to find a cause of their infant's premature delivery and medical problems. Health-care professionals, when telling mothers about the causes of their infants' medical problems, rarely mentioned more than complications of the pregnancy or their random occurrence. With this limited information, mothers formulated many theories of their own. One prominent causal ascription involved the mother's own behavior while she was pregnant, an attribution that has been termed behavioral self-blame. Included in the behavioral self-blame category were attributions to harmful habits, inadequate health behaviors, chronic phyical strain, hazardous physical activity, and the failure to adequately monitor prenatal care. Consistent with theory, mothers who made many of these self-attributions perceived more control over, and thought they could do more to prevent problems with, future pregnancies. Attributions to stable aspects of the self, primarily personality traits, did not help mothers view the future as more controllable.

At the same time, mothers who attributed the problem to their own behavior did not necessarily view the problem as having been avoidable. We speculated that this stance could attenuate some of the negative consequences of believing that their actions were causal. Although mothers who made these self-attributions more often experienced guilt over this perception, other evidence indicates that they were able to cope effectively with this emotion.

One attribution in particular was viewed by mothers as an avoidable cause: the perception of obstetric errors. In this and in previous studies, blaming others for victimizing events has almost always been associated with maladaptation. Several explanations of this relation were reviewed: (a) blaming others as a developmental diathesis, (b) the loss of personal control, (c) shattered illusions, and (d) the failure of vicarious control.

Chapter 6 moved from the analysis of cognitive adaptations to an inspection of mothers' strategies of coping with their child's intensive care. The hospitalization of a newborn on an intensive care unit elicits a spectrum of coping strategies. Our informants showed no clear consensus concerning the use of any specific coping strategy. Instead, they followed more than one approach, usually several, to contend with the stresses of this event. To some extent, their coping strategies were affected by facts such as their age and parity and were shaped by what they viewed as the most prominent stressor.

The highest proportions of mothers used strategies that involved seeking social support and finding meaning in the situation. These responses comprised slightly more than half the strategies mothers reported on the WOCC, and were volunteered by large proportions of mothers in response to our interview question. These mothers sought information, advice, and sympathy from others and tried to make valued changes in their life to achieve personal growth or to discover new faith or truth. Taking instrumental actions—a strategy that involves efforts toward problem solutions—comprised about 14% of mothers' overall coping efforts as measured by the coping checklist. Such active coping behaviors were also described by many mothers in the interview.

The last two coping strategies measured by the WOCC—minimizing and escaping—involve the regulation of emotional responses to this threatening event. Minimization, which accounted for 14% of mothers' coping strategies reported on the WOCC, involves deliberate efforts to ignore the problem or to view it in a less threatening way. Escaping the problem, which includes wishful thinking, avoidance of social contacts, and tension-reducing behaviors such as drinking and sleeping, represented 20% of mothers' coping efforts. It is more difficult to connect these strategies with what mothers described in the interview as their coping repertoire.

Although mothers who coped by trying to minimize the problem reported less emotional distress at NICU discharge, those who tried to escape or withdraw from the situation described their mood as more disturbed at this time. This may reflect the need of the more distressed mother to escape, or the intensification of distress the more the mother tries to withdraw. There were also certain threats posed by this crisis that may have prompted a desire to escape or were magnified by escapist behavior. In describing the crisis of their child's hospitalization, mothers who used more escapist coping more often mentioned the NICU environment itself as a threat. When the very setting in which their child was being treated is aversive, mothers might be expected to withdraw. As confirmation of this speculation, we also found that mothers who reported more escapist coping visited the NICU less often.

Escapist coping did not predict any long-term consequences for mothers or children when the mood disturbance accompanying this strategy was taken into account. Another coping strategy—taking instrumental actions —did predict mothers' well-being 18 months after discharge. Some researchers have shown that problem-focused coping solutions can be an effective way of alleviating the stressfulness of a threatening situation. Yet mothers who focused their coping efforts on coming up with solutions to the problem were more, not less, distressed 18 months after discharge, and this specific relation held up in the integrative analysis of all other predictors of mothers' longer term distress.

Why did these mothers exhibit greater subsequent distress? People who use more problem-directed coping usually appraise the stressful situation as more amenable to personal control (Lazarus & Folkman, 1984). But those mothers whose coping was more problem-focused did not actually perceive greater personal control over their child's outcome in the hospital. Thus, a problem-directed solution, which assumes a controllable outcome, did not afford these parents a sense of greater control. This mismatch between control expectancies, efforts to gain control through instrumental actions, and perceptions of actual control could engender long-term distress (Forsythe & Compas, 1987).

Furthermore, a control-oriented approach to coping with stressful events may, for all its virtues, draw the person's attention to the aversive aspects of the situation (Burger, 1989). It may also produce demoralization when problem solutions prove ineffective over the long run, as we suggested in Chapter 4. We might speculate further that if mothers who depended on problem solutions in the hospital continued to adopt this strategy in the months after discharge, they might later be more attentive to, and upset by, even minor problems in their child's health and development because they could not produce the desired outcome. Some support for this speculation was found in the fact that mothers who adopted this coping strategy were particularly likely to experience later distress when their child exhibited significant developmental delays or a neuromotor disability.

At the same time, these mothers provided more optimal home environments for their child. In particular, they scored higher on HOME Inventory subscales that reward a conscious effort to stimulate the child's development (i.e., the Provision of Appropriate Play Materials and the Maternal Involvement with Child subscales). These findings reveal that coping behaviors can affect or predict adaptation in different ways, depending on how one defines successful adaptation (Wortman, 1983).

Mothers whose coping was characterized by more efforts to minimize the problem reported more longer term distress, but only when their child was developmentally disabled. We surmise that efforts to minimize the severity of a stressful situation prove an ineffective coping strategy when the eventual severity of the outcome can no longer be ignored. Of the coping strategies we studied, only one—seeking meaning—predicted greater emotional well-being when the child's outcome was poor. Perhaps trying harder to find meaning, and doing so successfully, remains a source of comfort to mothers whose children fail to develop normally. In fact, mothers who had made a greater effort to find meaning in their child's hospitalization did agree more often with statements reflecting the discovery of a purpose in their plight. They were more likely to affirm a religious purpose, for example, "God selected me to give special care to this baby" and "This is one of the most important things that God will ever ask of me." But they also were more apt to believe that "This happened so that I could learn something important about myself." Thus, unlike the failure of problem-focused coping to increase a sense of control, efforts to find meaning appear to influence appraisals that suggest the discovery of meaning.

What's more, the children of mothers who had tried harder to find meaning had a better developmental outcome, an association that was not confounded by mothers' or childrens' characteristics assessed before hospital discharge. We have no ready explanation for this finding, but it does echo what we reported in chapter 3 about the poorer developmental outcomes of children whose mothers had found no benefits in the intensive care crisis.

In Chapter 7, our focus shifted to parents' interpersonal relationships and the role they played in the process of psychological adaptation. Mothers who were more distressed by their child's hospitalization and the burdens of the transition home expressed a greater need for help from other people. And those who found the support they needed appeared to be faring better during these times. This was especially true for the neediest mothers. Explanations of the relation between support and well-being in this and in other life crises are complex and require appreciation of dynamic and nonrecursive processes. Our findings raise important issues about the complex interdependencies of people's need for support, their satisfaction with support, and their well-being and between their coping strategies and the support they receive or fail to receive from others.

One interpretation of these findings is that mothers who were pleased with the assistance, information, and emotional support they secured from their family, friends, and the health professionals treating their child were better able to contend with the multifaceted demands of their child's hospitalization and its aftermath. Mothers who found themselves socially isolated during their baby's transition home were most likely to describe themselves as depressed, incompetent parents, unable to form a close relationship with their child. Path analysis revealed that mothers who had been more satisfied with their social support in the hospital were subsequently more attached to their child, which, in turn, was associated with less global distress a year later. That mothers' satisfaction with social support was a stronger predictor of their subsequent well-being when their child was developmentally disabled is yet another demonstration that support acts as a buffer against stress.

These mothers offered welcome insights into the ways in which relatives and friends can be helpful. Many stated their appreciation for others' expressions of concern and caring, efforts to reassure them of their coping abilities, and willingness to pitch in to make it easier for them to focus their attention on their baby in the hospital. Yet most mothers also described how well-meaning support gestures sometimes did more harm than good or how close friends and relatives distanced themselves.

We are intrigued by the findings that mothers found certain gestures helpful while others found the same gestures unhelpful. One such well-intentioned gesture is the attempt to supply a reason or purpose for this event. As we showed in Chapter 3, mothers' own inclination to appraise the newborn intensive care crisis as a purposeful event may aid their adaptation. But we suspect that this appraisal must be derived and cannot be effectively supplied. Watzlawick (1978) warned that the least helpful interventions are those that fail to consider the recipient's "language" or world view. Thus, parents who, for example, do not already believe that events are part of a divine plan are unlikely to appreciate well-intentioned interpretations of the birth of a premature infant as the will of God. All of this underscores the need for family and friends to be cautious in providing parents with positive appraisals of this crisis.

In Chapter 8, we explored the importance of social support, coping strategies, and cognitive adaptations in mothers' active memories of their child's hospitalization during the first and second years after hospital discharge. The findings reported in this chapter break new ground on the psychological meaning and adaptational significance of mothers' recurring memories of newborn intensive care. To begin, we revealed the complexity of mothers' memories of this stressful event. Most found themselves remembering both painful and pleasurable aspects of the hospital stay. Painful memories included how sick or close to death their baby had been, how hard it had been to adjust to this experience, problems they had encountered with their baby's physicians and nurses, and their sense of incompleteness as parents. Their pleasurable memories most often brought back to mind how supportive and competent the hospital staff had been, moments of closeness with their baby, and their feeling of awe for their baby's survival against what were thought to be great odds. All things considered, most mothers were grateful for these memories, declaring that they reinforced the personal growth they had witnessed in themselves, reminded them how precious their child was to them, helped them to appreciate their child's progress, and even kept them attuned to their child's special needs. Some mothers seemed to cherish these reminiscences so much that they would try to recapture their emotions by looking at photographs taken of the baby in the hospital or reading the thoughtful letters of well-wishers.

Many memories—both happy and sad—were evoked by events or environmental cues, including media reports on newborn intensive care and exposure to newborns and expectant mothers. As we had predicted, mothers' ability to find meaning in this crisis played a part in how they felt when they were reminded of that time. Those who had found a purpose in this event felt happier when their memories were triggered by events in the sixth month after discharge. And during the 18th month after discharge, pleasurable responses to reminders were more common among mothers who had found benefits or gains, whereas painful responses were more common among those who had not found benefits or gains. As we have already emphasized, these cognitive adaptations can help victims to overcome a sense of victimization and restore valued assumptions. They also appear, at least in this situation, to make a crisis less distressing when it comes back to mind.

Mothers who had reported problems in negotiating a satisfying partnership with their infant's care providers also encountered painful reminders in the sixth month after discharge. These mothers had described difficulties in obtaining desired control over their infant's care or in being kept adequately informed about their infant's treatment program. The distress evoked by these mothers' involuntary memories may be due, in part, to what they actually find themselves remembering about the hospital stay. More of these mothers did relate painful memories of difficult relationships with NICU personnel. Situational features of the crisis also had a short-term effect on mothers' painful response to reminders. Mothers of sicker, first-born infants were more likely to be subjected to painful reminders at 6 months, but not a year later.

Finally, we examined the intrusiveness of mothers' thoughts, emotions, and memories of the hospitalization and their efforts to avoid these thoughts, emotions, and reminders. We showed that intrusive and avoidant responses accompanied signs of maladaptation in both the first and second years after discharge. We also demonstrated that mothers who went to greater lengths to minimize the severity of the hospital crisis were less apt to experience intrusive memories and made fewer efforts to avoid them. This suggests that minimization may help some parents put the past behind them, although, as shown in Chapter 6, it may have undesirable consequences for mothers' well-being should the child become developmentally disabled. In contrast, those who had taken a more problem-directed approach in coping with their child's hospitalization were prone to more intrusive reminders and experienced increasing levels of intrusion over a year's time. The link between instrumental action coping and intrusive thoughts may be that both reflect a desire to master the threatening experience. Horowitz (1983), in his description of a stress response syndrome, views intrusive thoughts of stressful events as driven by a need to "repeat" the event in order to gain mastery over it.

In Chapter 9 we examined the crisis of newborn intensive care in the context of the marital relationship. Two types of comparisons were examined in this chapter. The first comparison was between husbands and their wives, that is, the concordances within couples. The second comparison was between mothers and fathers as a group. Marital partners were similar in their (a) appraisals of control over the infant's recovery in the hospital, (b) general expectations about the child's future health and development, (c) relative use of coping strategies that involved minimization, seeking meaning, and mobilizing support, (d) perceptions that the marital relationship had been improved by this crisis, and (e) satisfaction with their social support while their child was hospitalized. Spouses were not concordant on measures of psychological well-being, their use of coping strategies that involved taking instrumental actions and escaping the problem, and the perception that the hospitalization had caused marital problems.

Group differences between mothers and fathers can be summarized as follows: (a) mothers reported more mood disturbance at NICU discharge and 18 months later; (b) mothers perceived more personal control over their infant's recovery in the hospital, and were more likely to describe their efforts at providing social stimulation as efficacious; (c) mothers expressed more concerns about their child's future health and development, especially the fear that their child would become mentally retarded; (d) mothers' coping strategies included more attempts to escape the problem and greater absolute use of suport mobilization, whereas fathers' coping was characterized by greater relative use of instrumental actions and efforts to minimize the situation; (e) fathers were more apt to describe the marital relationship as being harmed by their child's hospitalization; and (f) fathers were more satisfied with the support they obtained from others during their child's hospitalization. Mothers and fathers were similar in their global psychological distress at 18 months, in their general expectancies of a positive outcome for their child, in their appraisals of the meaning of the crisis, and in their use of coping strategies that involved seeking meaning and seeking support.

We reasoned that gender differences in early mood disturbance might be due in part to the differential use of coping strategies that can magnify or alleviate disturbances in emotional well-being. Fathers, who used instrumental action coping more than mothers did before discharge, were less distressed when they adopted this strategy. On the other hand, mothers, who used escapist coping to a greater extent, were more distressed when they used this coping strategy. Although coping strategies played a role in each parent's own well-being, they did not figure in the well-being of one's partner. We speculated further that the lack of association between one partner's coping strategies and his or her partner's emotional adaptation could be due to differences in how partners evaluate their spouse's coping attempts. Although some spouses described adverse effects of their partner's coping style, others described benefits of the same coping strategies. This was seen most clearly in wives' differing appraisals of their husband's tendency to minimize the severity of the problem. Moreover, some spouses found differences in coping styles an added burden, whereas others saw them as advantageous.

Despite some fathers' observations that their wife had greater opportunities to secure support, fathers did not appear harmed by this imbalance. Many viewed as appropriate the greater attention paid to their wife's needs, fathers felt less need for support than mothers, and fathers' satisfaction with support did not figure in their well-being, as it did in their wife's adaptation. Finally, we showed that both mothers and fathers who cited benefits of this crisis for the marital relationship fared better in their longer term adaptation. What's more, mothers who described positive changes in their marriage were apt to have children who exhibited more positive developmental outcomes 18 months later.

Meeting Parents' Need for Support

According to crisis theory (Moos & Tsu, 1977), the emotional disequilibrium stemming from the hospitalization and transition home of medically fragile infants should make parents especially receptive to interventions that can improve their coping and adaptation. Formal support services could also compensate for gaps in the support these parents derive from family and friends. Helping professionals can supply many resources valued by people who are contending with stressful life events. Such resources include opportunities for the expression of disturbing feelings, information about the problem, advice and feedback about efficacious problem-solving strategies, and concrete aid and assistance.

The efficacy of supportive interventions for parents during the transition from hospital to home care of at-risk infants is beginning to be documented (Bustan & Sagi, 1984; Nurcombe, Howell, Rauh, Teti, Ruoff, & Brennan, 1984). Nonetheless, our own experience in providing and evaluating a supportive intervention program for mothers of medically fragile infants (Affleck et al., 1989), summarized below, raises key issues about the benefits and costs of professional helping.

A transitional consultation program was provided for a randomly selected half of the mothers in our study. These families were visited weekly by one of two nurses whose competencies included the ability to establish rapport; interviewing and listening skills; familiarity with newborn intensive care and developmental and medical disorders of infancy; knowledge of early developmental sequences, basic child care, and infant stimulation; ability to recognize atypical early development; working knowledge of habilitative therapies; and awareness of community services and early intervention programs.

This service was based on a consultation model of helping, as opposed to a parent-training or infant-curriculum model (see Affleck et al., 1982 for a discussion). The defining feature of this model is allowing mothers to dictate the specific topics for discussion within the broad guidelines of the consultant's views of the child's and family's best long-term interests. When a mother expressed no concerns or problems, the consultant played a more active role in raising issues for discussion, based on her assessment of the infant's characteristics and needs and observations of mother-infant interactions. Consultants' activities during home visits included listening to mothers' feelings and concerns, giving information on the characteristics of typical and atypical infants, observing and highlighting evidence of infants' development, mutual problem-solving, demonstrating therapeutic and caregiving procedures, and helping mothers to prepare for events and potential problems after termination of the problem 3 months after discharge.

We hypothesized that improvements in mothers' adaptation to the transition home as a result of participation in the support program would be greater for those who expressed a need for more support during the hospitalization. Consistent with this prediction, the effects of the program were conditional upon mothers' need for support. For mothers desiring a high level of support, the program engendered positive consequences for mothers' perceptions of control, sense of competence, and responsiveness to their infants. But for mothers who said they needed little support, participation in the program actually had negative effects on these outcomes.

The needs of mothers who had desired support may have been met more completely through the resources provided by the transitional consultation program. From additional evidence, including an inspection of the distribution of consultation activities for mothers needing more or less support, we reasoned that the needier mothers were more receptive to, and made more effective use of, the consultant's helping activities. We speculated further that some program participants with low support needs may have faced threats to their adaptation because the information imparted to them, which they did not actively seek, disrupted their positive view of their child's condition and caused them to question their competence as caregivers. We concluded from these findings that mothers would have been better served by being allowed to determine fully what they wanted, if anything, from this helping program. Merely knowing that professional support is available, even if it is never requested or used, could itself be a valued resource.

Implications for Helping

The evaluation of our transitional consultation program reveals the delicate dynamics of the helping process. Parents of medically fragile infants encounter many different helping professionals over the course of their child's infancy. Obviously, all interact with physicians, nurses, and allied professionals who work on the NICU. Pediatricians play a key role in caring for their child after discharge and many parents avail themselves of community-based early intervention services that put them in touch with early childhood special education teachers and other developmental specialists such as physical and occupational therapists. How can our findings improve the effectiveness of these professionals' dealings with parents of medically fragile infants and increase opportunities for genuinely helpful transactions between parents and professionals?

First, we urge helping professionals to question unwarranted assumptions about the coping process and patterns of adjustment to newborn intensive care and its aftermath. One conviction appearing in the clinical literature and underlying many professionals' preconceptions is that parents of handicapped or prematurely born infants pass through "stages" in their adaptation, typically moving from shock and denial to anger and guilt and finally to a stage of adjustment and acceptance. Blacher (1984) and Allen and Affleck (1985) argued that such staged progressions are not substantiated by empirical data, echoing Silver and Wortman's (1980) critique of the stage hypothesis of coping with bereavement and loss. The findings of this study defy any such categorization of stages of adjustment to the crisis of newborn intensive care. If anything, they document exceptional variability in parents' coping and adaptation. The danger is that when professionals hold stereotyped expectations of parental adjustment, their efforts to provide support are jeopardized and their relationship with parents will suffer. There is the risk of pushing parents in the direction of the next "stage" rather than working from the adaptational responses exhibited by each individual parent. We argue instead for the careful analysis of parents' coping responses and appraisals and respect for the many factors that account for the diversity of adjustment patterns.

Our findings document a rich array of coping responses to newborn intensive care. Helping professionals appear to welcome active problem-solving behaviors but may ignore other coping responses that appear to play a prominent role in longer term well-being, such as the search for meaning. Parents who are inclined to find solutions to problems need to be approached differently from those whose dominant coping response is to minimize the severity of the problem. In our view, neither coping strategy should be seen as superior and neither should be deliberately encouraged by helping professionals at the expense of the other. The importance of respecting individual differences is supported as well by what we learned of mothers' desire for control over their child's health care before discharge. Physicians and nurses working on NICUs should anticipate that parents will have varying needs for personal, vicarious, and participatory control and be prepared to respond differently to parents based on their assessment of these needs. Failure to accommodate those needs may not only make it more difficult for parents to contend with their child's hospitalization but can color their memories of this time years later.

Our findings should also help professionals to interpret better the psychological meaning of parents' appraisals of the newborn intensive care crisis and to respond more helpfully to their expressions. One example is the tendency of many parents to blame themselves for what happened to their baby. "Self-blame" is commonly thought to be a maladaptive and irrational response, but parents' tendency to blame themselves for their child's premature delivery may have adaptive consequences to the extent that it helps them regain a sense of personal control. Professionals might also be quick to dissuade parents from drawing comparisons about the severity of their infant's problems. In fact, some parents volunteered that their questions about other babies on the NICU were frowned upon by physicians and nurses. Comparison processes, or so it is feared, might undercut parents' "realistic" acceptance of the seriousness of the condition or, alternatively, might upset parents by exaggerating its severity. But the comparisons that parents make are predominantly to infants with more severe problems, and we doubt that these downward comparisons inhibit a realistic view of the problem. Instead they appear to supply comfort, especially during the first days of the crisis when other ways of coping may not yet be consolidated. Another example is mothers' expectation of control of their child's future health and development. This appraisal, which professionals might readily support as a way of motivating appropriate actions, may actually increase mothers' emotional distress and inhibit effective action.

Nothing about our findings, however, should be construed as a suggestion that professionals should manipulate attributions, comparisons, or other appraisals. As we learned from mothers' descriptions of unhelpful support gestures, a positive appraisal of the crisis supplied by another person, however well-intentioned, may not have the same effect as one that is self-generated. And although naturally occurring self-attributions may help infuse meaning into one's plight and buttress a sense of control, the same attribution suggested by another may elicit resentment. Conversely, efforts to discourage attributions, even if they appear harmful to the victim, can have untoward effects (Wortman, 1983). Until more is known, we advise practitioners to avoid the temptation to shape these beliefs.

What we have learned from our research program has led us to question our own assumptions about the *necessity* of professional help for the vast majority of parents of sick, premature infants. More than 10 years ago, we began our studies with the aim of documenting the impact of early intervention on these families' adjustment. We now know that professional assistance can help some of these families, namely those who are aware that they need and want help. But we also realized that other factors are far more robust determinants of family members' well-being and adjustment than is their use of professional support. Consequently, we became more and more impressed with what these families are able to accomplish without professional help. Other investigators studying adaptation to adversity are beginning to learn much the same thing. The following observations by Taylor (1983), whose research on coping with threatening events helped to frame our study, are a fitting conclusion to this book because they capture the spirit of our findings:

> One of the most impressive qualities of the human psyche is its ability to withstand severe personal tragedies successfully. Despite serious setbacks such as personal illness or the death of a family member, the majority of people facing such blows achieve a quality of life or level of happiness equivalent to or even exceeding their prior level of satisfaction. Not everyone readjusts, of course, but

most do, and furthermore they do so substantially on their own...They use their social networks and individual resources, and their apparent cure rate...is impressive even by professional standards...[T]he more [we] know about the human body, the more, not less miraculous it seems. The recuperative powers of the mind merit similar awe [pps. 1161 and 1171].

References

Abernathy, V. (1973). Social network and response to maternal role. *Journal of Sociology and the Family*, *3*, 86–92.

Abidin, R. (1983). *Parenting Stress Index*. Charlottesville, VA: Pediatric Psychology Press.

Affleck, G., Allen, D., McGrade, B., & McQueeney, M. (1982a). Maternal causal attributions at hospital discharge of high risk infants. *American Journal of Mental Deficiency*, *86*, 575–580

Affleck, G., Allen, D., McGrade, B., & McQueeney, M. (1982b). Home environments of developmentally disabled infants as a function of parent and child characteristics. *American Journal of Mental Deficiency*, *86*, 445–452.

Affleck, G., Allen, D., McGrade, B., & McQueeney, M. (1983). Maternal and child characteristics associated with mothers' perceptions of their developmentally disabled infants. *Journal of Genetic Psychology*, *142*, 171–180.

Affleck, G., Allen, D., Tennen, H., McGrade, B., & Ratzan, S. (1985). Causal and control cognitions in parent coping with a chronically ill child. *Journal of Social and Clinical Psychology*, *3*, 367–377.

Affleck, G., McGrade, B., Allen, D., & McQueeney, M. (1985). Mothers' beliefs about behavioral causes of their developmentally disabled infant's condition: What do they signify? *Journal of Pediatric Psychology*, *10*, 293–303.

Affleck, G., McGrade, B., McQueeney, M., & Allen, D. (1982). Promise of relationship-focused early intervention in developmental disabilities. *Journal of Special Education*, *16*, 413–430.

Affleck, G., Pfeiffer, C., Tennen, H., & Fifield, J. (1987). Attributional processes in rheumatoid arthritis patients. *Arthritis and Rheumatism*, *30*, 927–931.

Affleck, G., Pfeiffer, C., Tennen, H., & Fifield, J. (1988). Social support and psychosocial adjustment to rheumatoid arthritis: Quantitative and qualitative findings. *Arthritis Care and Research*, *1*, 71–77.

Affleck, G., & Tennen, H. (in press). Comparison processes and coping with serious medical disorders. In J. Suls & T.A. Wills (Eds.), *Social comparison: Contemporary theory and research*. Hillsdale, NJ: Erlbaum.

Affleck, G., Tennen, H., Allen D., & Gershman, K. (1986). Perceived social support and maternal adaptation during the transition from hospital to home care of high risk infants. *Infant Mental Health Journal*, *7*, 6–18.

Affleck, G., Tennen, H., Croog, S., & Levine, S. (1987a). Causal attribution, perceived benefits, and morbidity following a heart attack. *Journal of Consulting and Clinical Psychology*, *55*, 29–35.

Affleck, G., Tennen, H., Croog, S., & Levine, S. (1987b). Causal attribution, perceived control, and recovery from a heart attack. *Journal of Social and Clinical Psychology*, *5*, 339–355.

Affleck, G., Tennen, H., & Gershman, K. (1985). Cognitive adaptations to high risk infants: The search for meaning, mastery, and protection from future harm. *American Journal of Mental Deficiency*, *89*, 653–656.

Affleck, G., Tennen, H., Pfeiffer, C., & Fifield, J. (1987). Appraisals of control and predictability in adapting to a chronic disease. *Journal of Personality and Social Psychology*, *53*, 273–279.

Affleck, G., Tennen, H., Pfeiffer, C., & Fifield, J. (1988). Social comparisons in rheumatoid arthritis: Accuracy and adaptational significance. *Journal of Social and Clinical Psychology*, *6*, 219–234.

Affleck, G., Tennen, H., Pfeiffer, C., Fifield, J., & Rowe, J. (1987). Downward comparison and coping with serious medical problems. *American Journal of Orthopsychiatry*, *57*, 570–578.

Affleck, G., Tennen, H., Rowe, J., Roscher, B., & Walker, L. (1989). Effects of formal support on mothers' adaptation to the hospital-to-home transition of high risk infants: The benefits and costs of helping. *Child Development, 60,* 488–501.

Abert, S. (1977). Temporal comparison theory. *Psychological Review*, *84*, 485–503.

Allen, D., & Affleck, G. (1985). Are we stereotyping parents? A postscript to Blacher. *Mental Retardation*, *23*, 200–202.

Aldwin, C., & Revenson, T. (1987). Does coping help? A reexamination of the relation between coping and mental health. *Journal of Personality and Social Psychology*, *53*, 337–348.

Allen, D., McGrade, B., Affleck, G., & McQueeney, M. (1982). The predictive validity of neonatal intensive care nurses' judgments of the parent-child relationship: A nine-month follow-up. *Journal of Pediatric Psychology*, *7*, 125–134.

Averill, J. (1973). Personal control over aversive stimuli and its relationship to stress. *Psychological Bulletin*, *80*, 286–303.

Bader, D., Kamos, A., Lew, C., Platzker, A., Stabile, M., & Keens, T. (1987). Childhood sequelae of infant lung disease: Exercise and pulmonary function abnormalities after bronchopulmonary dysplasia. *Journal of Pediatrics*, *110*, 639–699.

Bandura, A. (1977). Self-efficacy: Toward a unifying theory of behavioral change. *Psychological Review*, *84*, 191–215.

Bard, M., & Sangrey, D. (1979). *The crime victim's book*. Boston: Beacon Press.

Barrera, M. (1981). Social support in the adjustment of pregnant adolescents: Assessment issues. In B. H. Gottlieb (Ed.), *Social networks and social support* (pp. 69–96). Beverly Hills: Sage.

Baum, A., Fleming, R., & Singer, J. (1983). Coping with victimization by technological disaster. *Journal of Social Issues*, *39*, 117–138.

Bayley, N. (1969). *Bayley Scales of Infant Development*. New York: Psychological Corporation.

Beckwith, L., & Cohen, S. (1984). Home enviornment and cognitive competence in preterm infants during the first 5 years. In A. Gottfried (Ed.), *Home environment and early cognitive development* (pp. 235–271). New York: Academic.

Belsky, J. (1983, April). *Social network contact and the transition to parenthood*. Paper presented at the Biennial Meeting of the Society for Research in Child Development, Detroit, MI.

Benfield, D., Leib, S., & Reuter, J. (1976). Grief response of parents after referral of the critically ill newborn to a regional center. *New England Journal of Medicine, 294*, 975–978.

Billings, A. G., & Moos, R. M. (1981). The role of coping responses and social resources in attenuating the stress of life events. *Journal of Behavioral Medicine, 4*, 139–157.

Blacher, J. (1984). Sequential stages of parental adjustment to the birth of a child with handicaps: Fact or artifact? *Mental Retardation, 22*, 55–68.

Blaney, P. (1986). Affect and memory: A review. *Psychological Bulletin, 99*, 229–246.

Bogdan, R., Brown, M., & Foster, S. (1982). Be honest but not cruel: Staff-parent communication on a neonatal unit. *Human Organization, 41*, 6–16.

Bolger, N., Delongis, A., Kessler, R., & Schilling, E. (1989). Effects of daily stress on negative mood. *Journal of Personality and Social Psychology, 57*, 808–818.

Boyd, I., Yeager, M., & McMillan, M. (1973). Personality styles in the postoperative course. *Psychosomatic Medicine, 35*, 131–134.

Breslau, N., Klein, N., & Allen, L. (1988). Very low birthweight: Behavioral sequelae at nine years of age. *Journal of the American Academy of Child Psychiatry, 27*, 605–612.

Brickman, P., Rabinowitz, V., Karuza, J., Coates, D., Cohn, E., & Kidder, L. (1982). Models of helping and coping. *American Psychologist, 37*, 368–384.

Briggs, D. (1985). *The impact on a family of having a newborn baby hospitalized on a newborn intensive care unit*. Unpublished doctoral dissertation, Brandeis University, Waltham, MA.

Brown, J., & Bakeman, R. (1980). Relationships of human mothers with their infants during the first year of life: Effects of prematurity. In R. Bell & W. Smotherman (Eds.), *Maternal influences and early behavior*. Holliswood, NY: Spectrum.

Bulman, R., & Wortman, C. (1977). Attributions of blame and coping in the "real world": Severe accident victims react to their lot. *Journal of Personality and Social Psychology, 35*, 351–363.

Burger, J. (1989). Negative reactions to increases in perceived personal control. *Journal of Personality and Social Psychology, 56*, 246–256.

Burgess, A., & Holstrom, L. (1979). *Rape: Crisis and recovery*. Bowie, MD: Brady.

Busch-Rossnagel, N., Peters, D., & Daly, M. (1984). Mothers of vulnerable and normal infants: More alike than different. *Family Relations, 33*, 149–154.

Bustan, D., & Sagi, A. (1984). Effects of early hospital-based intervention on mothers and their preterm infants. *Journal of Applied Developmental Psychology, 5*, 305–317.

Calame, A., Fawer, C., Claeys, Arrozola, S., Ducret, S., & Jaunin, L. (1986). Neurodevelopmental outcome and school performance of very low birth weight infants at 8 years of age. *European Journal of Pediatrics, 145*, 461–466.

Caldwell, B., & Bradley, R. (1984). *Home observation for measurement of the environment.* Unpublished manual, University of Arkansas, Little Rock.

Campbell, S., Breaux, A., Ewing, L., & Szumonowski, E. (1986). Correlates and predictors of hyperactivity and aggression: A longitudinal study of parent-referred problem preschoolers. *Journal of Abnormal Pscyhology*, *14*, 217–234.

Cella, D., Perry, S., Kulchycky, S., & Goodwin, C. (1988). Stress and coping in relatives of burn patients: A longitudinal study. *Hospital and Community Psychiatry*, *39*, 159–166.

Chesler, M., & Barbarin, O. (1984). Difficulties in providing help in a crisis: Relationships between parents of children with cancer and their friends. *Journal of Social Issues*, *40*, 113–134.

Cohen, S., & Parmelee, A. (1983). Prediction of five-year Stanford Binet scores in preterm infants. *Child Development*, *54*, 1242–1253.

Cohen, S., Parmelee, A., Sigman, M., & Beckwith, L. (1988). Antecedents of school problems in children born preterm. *Journal of Pediatric Psychology*, *13*, 493–508.

Cohen, S., & McKay, G. (1984). Social support, stress and the buffering hypothesis: A theoretical analysis. In A . Brown, J. E. Stinger, & S. E. Taylor (Eds.), *Handbook of psychology and health* (Vol. 4). Hillsdale, N J: Erlbaum⊕

Coyne, J., Aldwin, C., & Lazarus, R. (1981). Depression and coping in stressful episodes. *Journal of Abnormal Psychology*, *90*, 439–477.

Coyne, J., & DeLongis, A. (1986). Going beyond social support: The role of social relationships in adaptation. *Journal of Consulting and Clinical Psychology*, *54*, 454–460.

Crnic, K. Greenberg, M., Ragozin, A., Robinson, N., & Basham, R. (1983). Effects of stress and social support on mothers and premature and full-term infants. *Child Development*, *54*, 209–217.

Crnic, K., Greenberg, M., & Slough, N. (1986). Early stress and social support influences on mothers' and high risk infants' functioning in late infancy. *Infant Mental Health Journal*, *7*, 19–33.

Crnic, K., Greenberg, M., Robinson, N., & Ragozin, A. (1984). Maternal stress and social support: Effects on the mother-infant relationship from birth to eighteen months. *American Journal of Orthopsychiatry*, *54*, 224–235.

Cutrona, C., & Troutman, B. (1986). Social support, infant temperament, and parenting self-efficacy: A mediational model of postpartum depression. *Child Development*, *57*, 1507–1518.

DeFrain, J. (1986). *Stillborn: The invisible death.* Lexington, MA: D.C. Heath and Company.

Derogatis, L. (1977). *SCL-90: Administration, scoring and procedures manual for the revised version.* Baltimore: Clinical Biometrics Research Series.

DeVellis, R., Holt, K., Renner, B., Blalock, S., Blanchard, L., Cook, H., Klotz, M., Mikow, V., & Harring, K. (in press). The relationship of social comparison to rheumatoid arthritis symptoms and affect. *Basic and Applied Social Psychology.*

DiVitto, B., & Goldberg, S. (1979). The effects of newborn medical status on early parent-infant interaction. In T. Field (Ed.), *Infants born at risk* (pp. 311–332). New York, NY: Spectrum.

Dunkel-Schetter, C. (1984). Social support and cancer: Findings based on patients interviews and their implications. *Journal of Social Issues*, *40*, 77 98.

Dunkel-Schetter, C., Folkman, S., & Lazarus, R. (1987). Correlates of social support receipt. *Journal of Personality and Social Psychology, 53,* 71–80.

Dunst, C., & Trivette, C. (1987, April). *Social Support and positive functioning in families of developmentally disabled infants.* Paper presented at the Biennial Meeting of the Society for Research in Child Development, Baltimore, MD.

Dunst, C., Trivette, C., & Cross, A. (1985). Mediating influences of social support: Personal, family, and child outcomes. *American Journal of Mental Deficiency, 90,* 403–417.

Ellison. P, (1984). Neurologic development of the high risk infant. *Clinics in Perinatology, 11,* 41–58.

Escalona, S. (1982). Babies at double hazard: Early development of infants at biological and social risk. *Pediatrics, 70,* 670–676.

Felton, B., & Revenson, T. (1984). Coping with chronic illness: A study of illness controllability and the influence of coping strategies on psychological adjustment. *Journal of Consulting and Clinical Psychology, 52,* 343–353.

Felton, B., Revenson, T., & Hinrichsen, G. (1984). Stress and coping in the explanatiion of psychological adjustment among chronically ill adults. *Social Science and Medicine, 18,* 889–898.

Fenichel, O. (1945). *The psychoanalytic theory of neurosis,* New York: W.W. Norton.

Festinger, L. (1954). A theory of social comparison processes. *Human Relations, 7,* 117–140.

Field, T., Sostek, A., Goldberg, S., & Schuman, H. (Eds.) (1979). *Infants born at risk: Behavior and development.* New York: Medical and Scientific Books.

Fiore, J., Becker, J., & Coppel, D. (1983). Social network interactions: Buffer or stress? *American Journal of Community Psychology, 11,* 423–440.

Fleishman, J. (1984). Personality characteristics and coping patterns. *Journal of Health and Social Behavior, 25,* 229–244.

Folkman, S. & Lazarus, R. (1980). An analysis of coping in a middle-aged community sample. *Journal of Health and Social Behavior, 21,* 219–239.

Folkman, S., & Lazarus, R. (1985). If it changes it must be a process: Study of emotion and coping during three stages of a college examination: *Journal of Personality and Social Psychology, 48,* 150–170.

Forsythe, C., & Compas, B. (1987). Interaction of cognitive appraisals of stressful events and coping: Testing the goodness of fit hypothesis. *Cognitive Therapy and Research, 11,* 473–485.

Freud, S. (1923). *The ego and id.* London: Hogarth.

Frey, D., Rogner, O., Schuler, M., & Korte, C. (1985). Psychological determinants in the convalescence of accident patients. *Basic and Applied Social Psychology, 6,* 317–328.

Garcia-Coll, G. (1983, April). *The effects of child care support, SES, education, and life stress on the home environment of adolescent mothers.* Paper presented at the Biennial Meeting of the Society for Research in Child Development, Detroit, MI.

Gleuckauf, R., & West, S. (1981, August). *The uncertainties of coping with epilepsy.* Paper presented at the annual meeting of the American Psychological Association, Los Angeles, CA.

Goldberg, S. (1979). Premature birth: Consequences for the parent-infant relationship. *American Scientist, 67,* 214–220.

Gotay, C. (1985). Why me? Attributions and adjustment by cancer patients and their mates at two stages in the disease process. *Social Science and Medicine*, *20*, 825–831.

Gottman, M., & Levenson, R. (1988). The social psychophysiology of marriage. In P. Noller & M. Fitzpatrick (Eds.), *Perspectives on marital interaction* (pp. 182–200). Philadelphia: Multilingual Matters.

Gowan, J., Appelbaum, M., & Johnson-Martin, N. (1987, April). *Predictors of distress and feelings of parenting competence in mothers of delayed and nondelayed infants*. Paper presented at the Biennial Meeting of the Society for Research in Child Development, Baltimore, MD.

Green, M., & Solnit, A. (1964). Reactions to the threatened loss of a child: A vulnerable child syndrome. *Pediatrics*, *34*, 58–66.

Greenberg, M., & Crnic, K. (1988). Longitudinal predictors of developmental status and social interaction in premature and full-term infants at age two. *Child Development*, *59*, 554–570.

Gribbins, R., & Marshall, R. (1984). Stress and coping strategies of nurse managers in the NICU. *Journal of Perinatology*, *1*, 268–271.

Gunn, T., Lepore, E., & Outerbridge, E. (1983). Outcome at school age after mechanical ventilation. *Developmental Medicine and Child Neurology*, *25*, 305–314.

Heppner, P., Reeder, B., & Larson, L. (1983). Cognitive variables associated with personal problem solving appraisal: Implications for counseling. *Journal of Counseling Psychology*, *30*, 537–545.

Hertzig, M., & Mittleman, M. (1984). Temperament in low birthweight children. *Merrill-Palmer Quarterly*, *30* 201–211.

Herzog, J. (1979). Disturbances in parenting high-risk infants. In T. Field (Ed.), *Infants born at risk: Behavior and development* (pp. 357–364). New York, NY: Spectrum.

Horowitz, M. (1983). Psychological response to serious life events. In S. Breznitz (Ed.), *The denial of stress* (pp. 129–159). New York: International Universities Press.

Horowitz, M., Wilner, N., & Alvarez, W. (1979). Impact of event scale: A measure of subjective stress. *Psychosomatic Medicine*, *41*, 209–218.

How, E., Bill, J., & Sykes, D. (1988). Very low birthweight: A long-term developmental impairment. *International Journal of Behavioral Development*, *11*, 37–67.

Janoff-Bulman, R. (1979). Characterological versus behavioral self-blame: Inquiries into depression and rape. *Journal of Personality and Social Psychology*, *37*, 1798–1809.

Janoff-Bulman, R. (1989). The benefits of illusions, the threat of disillusionment, and the limitations of inaccuracy. *Journal of Social and Clinical Psychology*, *8*, 158–175.

Janoff-Bulman, R., & Frieze, I. (1983). A theoretical perspective for understanding reactions to victimization. *Journal of Social Issues*, *39*, 1–17.

Jeffcoate, J., Humphrey, M., & Lloyd, L. (1979). Role perception and response to stress in fanthers and mothers after pre-term delivery. *Social Science and Medicine*, *13*, 139–145.

Kenny, D. (1975). Cross-lagged panel correlation: A test for spuriousness. *Psychological Bulletin*, *82*, 887–903.

Kerlinger, F., & Pedhazur, E. (1973). *Multiple regression in behavioral research*. New York. Holt, Rinehart, and Winston.

Kernberg, O. (1975). *Borderline conditions and pathological narcissism* New York: Jason Aronson.

Kiecolt-Glaser, J., & Williams, D. (1987). Self-blame, compliance, and distress among burn patients. *Journal of Personality and Social Psychology, 53*, 187–193.

Kim, Y., Wheeler, W., Logmate, J., & Wohl, M. (1988). Longitudinal study of function in children following bronchopulmonary dysplasia. *American Reveiw of Respiratory Disease, 137*, 13.

Klein, M. (1964). *Contributions to psychoanalysis: 1920–1945.* New York: McGraw-Hill.

Klein, N., Hack, M., Gallagher, J., & Fanaroff, A. (1985). Preschool performance of children with normal intelligence who were very low birthweight infants. *Pediatrics, 75*, 531–537.

Klinger, E. (1975). Consequences of commitment to and disengagement from incentives. *Psychological Review, 82*, 1–25.

Kohut, H. (1977). *The restoration of the self.* New York: International Universities Press.

Kopp, C., & Kaler, S. (1989). Risk in infancy: Origins and implications. *American Psychologist, 44*, 224–230.

Lambert, V. (1981). *Factors affecting psychological well-being in women with reheumatoid arthritis*: Unpublished doctoral dissertation, University of California, San Francisco, CA.

Landry, S., Chapieski, L., Fletcher, J., & Denson, S. (1988). Three-year outcomes for low birth weight infants: Differential effects of early medical complications. *Journal of Pediatric Psychology, 13*, 317–327.

Langer, E. (1975). The illusion of control. *Journal of Personality and Social Psychology, 32*, 311–328.

Langer, E., & Rodin, J. (1976). The effects of choice and enhanced personal responsibility: A field experiment in an institutional setting. *Journal of Personality and Social Psychology, 34* 191–198

Lazarus, R., & Folkman, S. (1984). *Stress, appraisal and coping.* New York: Springer.

Lefebrve, F., Bard, H., Veilleux, A., & Martel, C. (1988). Outcome at school age of children with birthweight of 1000 grams or less. *Developmental Medicine and Child Neurology, 30*, 170–180.

Lehman, D., Ellard, J., & Wortman, C. (1986). Social support for the bereaved: Recipients' and providers' perspectives on what is helpful. *Journal of Consulting and Clinical Psychology, 54*, 438–446.

Lehman, D., Wortman, C., & Williams, A. (1987). Long-term effects of losing a spouse or child in a motor vehicle crash. *Journal of Personality and Social Psychology, 52*, 208–213.

Levy-Schiff, R., Sharir, H., & Mogilner, M. (1987). Mother-and father-preterm infant relationship in the hospital preterm nursery. *Child Development, 60*, 93–102.

Lindgren, S., Harper, D., & Blackman, J. (1986). Environmental influences and perinatal risk factors in high risk children. *Journal of Pediatric Psychology, 11*, 531–547.

Lloyd, B. (1984). Outcome of very low birthweight babies from Wolverhampton. *Lancet, 2*, 739–741.

Lorr, M., & McNair, D. (1982) *Profile of Mood States-B.* San Diego: Educational and Industrial Testing Service.

Lowery, B., Jacobsen, B., & Murphy, B. (1983). An exploratory investigation of causal thinking of arthritics. *Nursing Research*, *25*, 157–162.

Lyman, R., Wurtele, S., & Wilson, D. (1985). Psychological effects on parents of home and hospital apnea monitoring. *Journal of Pediatric Psychology*, *10*, 439–448.

Macey, T., Harmon, R., & Easterbrooks, M. (1987). Impact of premature birth on the development of the infant in the family. *Journal of Consulting and Clinical Psychology*, *55*, 846–852.

Manne, S., & Zautra, A. (1989). Spouse criticism and support: Their association with coping and psychological adjustment among women with rheumatoid arthritis. *Journal of Personality and Social Psychology*, *56*, 608–617.

Marshall, R,. & Kasman, C. (1980). Burnout in the neonatal intensive care unit. *Pediatrics*, *65*, 1161–1165.

McCormick, M. (1989). Long-term follow-up of infants discharged from neonatal intensive care units. *Journal of the American Medical Association*, *261*, 1767–1772.

McCormick, M., Stemmler, M., Bernbaum, J., & Farran, A. (1986). The very low birth weight transport goes home: Impact on the family. *Journal of Developmental and Behavioral Pediatrics*, *7*, 217–223.

McGehee, L., & Eckerman, C. (1983). The preterm infant as social partner: Responsive but unreadable. *Infant Behavior and Development*, *6*, 461–470.

McKinney, B., & Peterson, R. (1984). Parenting Stress Index. In D. Keyser & R. Sweetland (Eds.), *Test critiques*: *Vol 1* (pp. 504–510). Kansas City, MO: Test Coporation of America.

McNeil, T., Weigerink, R., & Dozier, J. (1970). Pergnancy and birth complications in the births of seriously disturbed children. *Journal of Nervous and Mental Diseases*, *151*, 24–34.

Meissner, W. (1978). *The paranoid press*. New York: Jason-Aronson.

Mendola, R., Tennen, H., Affleck, G., McCann, L., & Fitzgerald, T. (in press). Appraisal and adaptation among women with impaired fertility. *Cognitive Therapy and Research*.

Meyer, B., & Taylor, S. (1986). Adjustment to rape. *Journal of Personality and Social Psychology*, *51*, 1226–1234.

Miller, S. (1980). Why having control reduces stress: If I can stop the roller coaster, I don't want to get off. In J. Barber & M. Seligman (Eds.), *Human helplessness*: *Theory and applications* (pp. 71–95). New York: Academic Press.

Mintzer, D., Als, H., Tronick, E., & Brazelton, T. (1985). Parenting an infant with a birth defect: The regulation of self-esteem. *Zero to Three*, *5*, 1–8.

Moos, R., & Tsu, V. (1977). The crisis of physical illness: An overview. In R. Moos (Ed.), *Coping with physical illness* (pp. 3–22). New York: Plenum.

Mueller, P., & Major, B. (1989). Self-blame, self-efficacy, and adjustment to abortion. *Journal of Personality and Social Psychology*, *57*, 1059–1068.

Nicassio, P., Wallston, K., Callahan, L., Herbert, M., & Pincus, T. (1985). The measurement of helplessness in rheumatoid arthritis: The development of the Arthritis Helplessness Index. *Journal of Rheumatology*, *12*, 462–467.

Nielson, W., & McDonald, M. (1988). Attributions of blame and coping following spinal cord injury: Is self-blame adaptive? *Journal of Social and Clinical Psychology*, *7*, 163–175.

Nurcombe, B., Howell, D., Rauh, V., Teti, D., Ruoff, R., & Brennan, J. (1984). An intervention program for mothers of low birthweight infants. *Journal of the American Academy of Child Psychiatry*, *23*, 319–325.

O'Grady, D., & Metz, R. (1987). Resilience in children at high risk for psychological disorder. *Journal of Pediatric Psychology*, *12*, 3–23.

Page, M., Becker, J., & Coppel, D. (1985). Loss of control, self-blame, and depression: An investigation of spouse caregivers of Alzheimer's disease patients. *Journal of Abnormal Psychology*, *94*, 169–182.

Palfrey, J., Levine, M., Walker, D., & Sullivan, M. (1985). The emergence of attention deficits in early childhood. *Developmental and Behavioral Pediatrics*, *6*, 339–348.

Parker, J., McCrae, C., Smarr, K., Beck, N., Frank, R., Anderson, S., & Walker, S. (1988). Coping strategies in rheumatoid arthritis. *Journal of Rheumatology*, *15*, 1376–1383.

Parkes, C. (1975). What becomes of redundant world models? A contribution to the study of adaptation to change. *British Journal of Medical Psychology*, *48*, 131–137.

Parkes, K. (1984). Locus of control, cognitive appraisal, and coping in stressful episodes. *Journal of Personality and Social Psychology*, *46*, 655–668.

Parks, P., & Lenz, E. (1987, April). *Stress and support for mothers and infants*. Paper presented at the Biennial Meeting of the Society for Research in Child Development, Baltimore, MD.

Pascoe, J., Loda, G., Jeffries, V., & Earp, J. (1981). The association between mothers' social support and the provision of stimulation to their children. *Journal of Developmental and Behavioral Pediatrics*, *2*, 15–19.

Pearlin, L. I., & Schooler, C. (1978). The structure of coping. *Journal of Health and Social Behavior*, *19*, 2–21.

Pederson, D., Bento, S., Chance, G., Evans, B., & Fox, A. (1987). Maternal emotional responses to preterm birth. *American Journal of Orthopsychiatry*, *57*, 15–21.

Pederson, D., Evans, B., Chance, G., Bento, A., & Fox, A. (1988). Predictors of one-year developmental status in low birth weight infants. *Developmental and Behavioral Pediatrics*, *9*, 287–292.

Perloff, L. (1983). Perceptions of vulnerability to victimization. *Journal of Social Issues*, *39*, 41–61.

Perrin, E., West, P., & Culley, B. (1989). Is my child normal yet? Correlates of vulnerability. *Pediatrics*, *83*, 355–363.

Peterson, C., & Seligman, M. (1984). Causal explanations as a risk factor for depression: Theory and evidence. *Psychological Review*, *91*, 347–374.

Phibbs, C., Williams. R., & Phibbs, R. (1981). Newborn risk factors and costs of neonatal intensive care. *Pediatrics*, *68*, 313–321.

Philipp, C. (1983). The role of recollected anxiety in parental adaptation to low birthweight infants. *Child Psychiatry and Human Development*, *13*, 239–248.

Philips, L. (1968). *Human adaptation and its failures*. New York: Academic Press.

Plunkett, J., Meisels, S., & Stiefel, G. (1986). Patterns of attachment among perterm infants of varying biological risk. *Journal of the American Academy of Child Psychiatry*, *25*, 794–798.

Procidano, M. (1985). Home observation for measurement of the environment. In

D. Keyser & R. Sweetland (Eds.), *Test critiques: Vol. II* (pp. 337–346). Kansas City, MO: Test Corporation of America.

Raugh, V., & Achenbach, T. (1987, April). *Correlates of cognitive development and behavior problems and among low children from birth to four.* Paper presented at the Biennial Meeting of the Society for Research in Child Development, Baltimore, MD.

Raugh, V., Achenbach, T., Nurcombe, B., Howell, C., & Teti, D. (1988). Minimizing adverse effects of low birthweight: Four-year results of an early intervention program. *Child Development, 59,* 544–553.

Reid, D. (1984). Participatory control and the chronic illness adjustment process. In H. Lefcourt (Ed.), *Reasearch with the locus of control contruct: Extensions and limitations* (Vol. 3, pp. 361–389). New York: Academic Press.

Revenson, T. (1981). Coping with loneliness: *The impact of causal attributions. Personality and Social Psychology Bulletin, 7,* 565–571.

Revenson, T., & Felton, B. (1989). Disability and coping as predictors of psychological adjustment to rheumatoid arthritis. *Journal of Consulting and Clinical Psychology, 57,* 344–348.

Revenson, T., Wollman, C., & Felton, B. (1983). Social supports as stress buffers for adult cancer patients. *Psychosomatic Medicine, 45,* 321–331.

Rook, K. (1984). The negative side of social interaction: Impact on psychological well-being. *Journal of Personality and Social Psychology, 46,* 1097–1108.

Ross, G., Schechner, S., & Frayer, W. (1982). Perinatal and neurobehavioral predictors of one-year outcomes in infants < 1500 grams. *Seminars in Perinatology, 6,* 288–293.

Rothbaum, F., Weisz, J., & Snyder, S. (1982). Changing the world and changing the self: A two-process model of preceived control. *Journal of Personality and Social Psychology, 42,* 5–37.

Rowe, J., Clyman, R., Green, C., Mikkelsen, C., Haight, J., & Ataide, L. (1978). Follow-up of families who experience a perinatal death. *Pediatrics, 62,* 166–170.

Rutter, M. (1981). Stress, coping, and development: Some issues and some questions. *Journal of Child Psychology and Psychiatry, 22,* 323–356.

Rutter, M. (1988). Epidemiological approaches to developmental psychology. *Archives of General Psychiatry, 45,* 486–495.

Scheier, M., & Carver, C. (1987). Dispositional optimism and physical well-being: The infleunce of generalized outcome expectancies on health. *Journal of Personality, 55,* 169–210.

Scheppele, K., & Bart, P. (1983). Through women's eyes: Defining danger in the wake of sexual assault. *Journal of Social Issues, 39,* 63–80.

Schulz, R., & Decker, S. (1985). Long-term adjustment to physcial disability : The role of social support, perceived control, and self-blame. *Journal of Personality and Social Psychology, 48,* 1162–1172.

Seligman, M. (1975). *Helplessness: On depression, development, and death.* San Francisco, CA: Freeman.

Sell, E., Gaines, J., Gluckman, C., & Williams, E. (1985). Early identification of learning problems in neonatal intensive care graduates. *American Journal of Diseases in Children, 139,* 460–463.

Shaver, K. (1970). Defensive attribution: Effects of severity and relevance on the responsibility assigned for an accident. *Journal of Personality and Social Psy-*

chology, 14, 101–113.

Shumaker, S., & Brownell, A. (1984). Toward a theory of social support: Closing conceptual gaps. *Journal of Social Issues, 40*, 11–36.

Siegel, L. (1982). Reproductive, Perinatal, and environmental variables as predictors of development of preterm (<1501 grams) and full-term children at five years. *Seminars in Perinatology, 6*, 274–279.

Siegel, L., Saigal, S., Rosenbaum, P., Morton, R., Young, A., Berenbaum, S., & Stoskopf, B. (1982). Predictors of development in preterm and full-term infants: A model for detecting the "at-risk" child. *Journal of Pediatric Psychology, 7*, 135–148.

Silcock, A. (1984). Crises in parents of prematures: An Australian study. *British Journal of Developmental Psychology, 2*, 257–268.

Silver, R., Boon, C., & Stones, M. (1983). Searching for meaning in misfortune: Making sense of incest. *Journal of Social Issues, 39*, 81–102.

Silver, R., & Wortman, C. (1980). Coping with undesirable life events. In J. Garver & M. Seligman (Eds.), *Human helplessness: Theory and applications*. New York: Academic Press.

Sirigano, S., Kozinn, B., & Lachman, M. (1987, April). *The role of social support stress, and experience in the transition to parenthood*, Paper presented at the Biennial Meeting of the Society for Research in Child Development, Baltimore, MD.

Solomon, L., & Rothblum, E. (1986). Stress, coping, and social support in women. *Behavior Therapist, 9*, 199–204.

Sparrow, S., Balla, D., & Cicchetti, D. (1984). *Vineland Adaptive Behavior Scales*. Circel Pines, MN: American Guidance Service.

Spinetta, L., Swarner, J., & Sheposh, J. (1981). Effective parental coping following the death of a child with cancer. *Journal of Pediatric Psychology, 6*, 251–263.

Stanton, A., Tennen, H., Affleck, G., & Mendola, R. (1990). *Cognitive appraisal, coping processes, and adjustment to infertility*. Manuscript submitted for publication.

Stein, R., Gortmaker, S., Perrin, E., Perrin, J., Pless, I., Walker, D., & Weitzman, M. (1987). Severity of illness: Concepts and measurements. *Lancet, 2*, 1506–1509.

Steiner, I. (1979). Three kinds of reported choice. In L. Perlmuter & R. Monty (Eds.), *Choice and perceived control* (pp. 17–27). Hillsdale, NJ: Erlbaum.

Stone, A., Helder, L., & Schneider, M. (1988). Coping with stressful events: Coping dimensions and issues. In L. Cohen (Ed.), *Life events and psychological functioning; Theoretical and methodological issues* (pp. 182–210). Newbury Park, CA: Sage Publications.

Stone, A., & Neale, L. (1984). New measure of daily coping: Development and preliminary results. *Journal of Personality and Social Psychology, 46*, 892–906.

Sullivan, H. (1956). *Clinical studies in psychiatry*. New York: Norton.

Suls, J. (1977). Social comparison theory and research: An overview from 1945. In J. Suls & R. Miller (Eds.), *Social comparison processes: Theoretical and empirical perspectives* (pp. 1–20). Washington, DC: Hemisphere.

Suls, J., & Mullen, B. (1982). From the cradle to the grave: Comparison and self-evaluation across the life span. In J. Suls (Ed.), *Psychological perspectives on the self* (Vol. I) (pp. 97–125). Hillsdale, NJ: Erlbaum.

Taylor, S. (1983). Adjustment to threatening events: A theory of cognitive adapation. *American Psychologist*, *38*, 624–630.

Taylor, S., & Brown, J. (1988). Illusion and well-being: A social-psychological perspective on mental health. *Psychological Bulletin*, *103*, 193–210.

Taylor, S., Lichtman, R., & Wood, J. (1984). Attributions, beliefs about control, and adjustment to breast cancer. *Journal of Personality and Social Psychology*, *46*, 489–502.

Taylor, S., Wood, J., & Lichtman, R. (1983). It could be worse: Selective evaluation as a response to victimization. *Journal of Social Issues*, *39*, 19–40.

Taylor, S., & Lobel, M. (in press). Social comparison activity under threat: Downward evaluation and upward contacts. *Psychological Review*.

Tennen, H., & Affleck, G. (in press). Blaming others for threatening events. *Psychological Bulletin*.

Tennen, H., & Affleck, G., Allen, D., McGrade, B., & Ratzan, S. (1984). Causal attributions and coping with insulin-dependent diabetes. *Basic and Applied Social Psychology*, *5*, 131–142.

Tennen, H., Affleck, G., & Herzbeger, S. (1985). The Revised Symptom Checklist-90. In R. Sweetland & D. Keyser (Eds.), *Test critiques*: *Vol. III* (pp. 583–594). Kansas City, MO: Test Cooporation of America.

Tennen, H., Affleck, G., & Gershman, K. (1986). Self-blame in parents of infants with perinatal complications: The role of self-protective motives. *Journal of Personality and Social Psychology*, *50*, 690–696.

Tennen, H., Affleck, G., & Mendola, R. (in press). Coping with smell and taste disorders. In T. Getchell, R. Doty, L. Bartoshuk, & J. Snow, *Smell and taste in health and disease*. New York: Raven Press.

Tennen, H., & Herzberger, S. (1985a). Ways of Coping Scale. In D. Keyser & R. Sweetland (Eds.), *Test Critiques*: *Vol. III* (pp. 686–697). Kansas City, MO: Test Corporation of America.

Tennen, H., & Herzberger, S. (1985b). Impact of Event Scale. In D. Keyser & R. Sweetland (Eds.), *Test critiques*: *Vol. III* (pp. 358–366). Kansas City, MO: Test Corporation of America.

Thompson, S. (1981). Will it hurt less if I can control it? A complex answer to a simple question. *Psychological Bulletin*, *90*, 89–101.

Thompson, S. (1985). Finding positive meaning in a stressful event and coping. *Basic and Applied Social Psychology*, *6*, 279–295.

Thompson, S., & Janigian, A. (1988). Life schemes: A framework for understanding the search for meaning. *Journal of Social and Clinical Psychology*, *7*, 260–280.

Timko, C., & Janoff-Bulman, R. (1985). Attributions, vulnerability, and psychological adjustment: The case of breast cancer. *Health Psychology*, *4*, 521–546.

Towle, P., Bach, M., Hauck, D., Katzenstein, M., Dweck, H., & Crimmins, D. (1987, April). *Preschool behavior problems of nicu graduates*. Paper presented at the Biennial Meeting of the Society for Research in Child Development, Baltimore, MD.

Trause, M., & Kramer, L. (1983). The effects of premature birth on parents and their relationship. *Developmental Medicine and Child Neurology*, *25*, 459–465.

Trout, M. (1983). Birth of a sick or handicapped infant: Impact on the family. *Child Welfare*, *62*, 337–348.

Vaillant, G. (1977). *Adaptation to life*. Boston: Little, Brown.

Vingerhoets, A., & Flohr, P. (1984). Type A behaviour and self-reports of coping preferences. *British Journal of Medical Psychology*, *57*, 15–21.

Vitaliano, P., Maiuro, R., Russo, J., & Becker, J. (1985). Raw versus relative scores in the assessment of coping strategies. *Journal of Behavioral Medicine*, *10*, 1–18.

Walster, E. (1966). Assignment of responsibility for an accident. *Journal of Personality and Social Psychology*, *3*, 73–79.

Walwork, E., & Ellison, P. (1985). Follow-up of families of neonates in whom life support was withdrawn. *Clinical Pediatrics*, *24*, 14–20.

Watzlawick, P. (1978). *The language of change*. New York: Basic Books.

Weissman, A., & Worden, J. (1976). The existential plight in cancer: Significance of the first 100 days. *International Journal of Psychiatry in Medicine*, *7*, 1–15.

Werner, E., & Smith, R. (1982). *Vulnerable but invincible: A study of resilient children*. San Francisco, CA: McGraw-Hill.

Westbrook, M., Gething, L., & Bradbury, B. (1987). Beliefs in ability to control chronic illness: Associated evaluations and medical experiences. *Australian Psychologist*, *22*, 203–218.

Wethington, E., McLeod, J., & Kessler, R. (1987). The importance of life events for explaining sex differences in psychological distress. In R. Barnett, L. Biener, & G. Baruch (Eds.), *Gender and stress* (pp. 144–156). New York: Free Press.

Wills, T.A. (1981). Downward comparison principles in social psychology. *Psychological Bulletin*, *90*, 245–271.

Wills, T.A. (1987). Downward comparison as a coping mechanism. In C.R. Snyder & C. Ford (Eds.), *Coping with negative events: Clinical and social psychological perspectives* (pp. 243–268). New York: Plenum.

Witenberg, S., Blanchard, E., Suls, J., Tennen, H., McCoy, G., & McGoldrick, M. (1983). Perceptions of control and causality as predictors of compliance and coping in hemodialysis. *Basic and Applied Social Psychology*, *4*, 319–336.

Wood, J., Taylor, S., & Lichtman, R. (1985). Social comparison in adjustment to breast cancer. *Journal of Personality and Social Psychology*, *49*, 1169–1183.

Woodruff, D., & Birren, J. (1972). Age changes and cohort differences in personality. *Developmental Psychology*, *6*, 252–259.

Wortman, C. (1983). Coping with victimization: Conclusions and implications for future research. *Journal of Social Issues*, *39*, 197–223.

Wortman, C., & Dunkel-Schetter, C. (1979). Interpersonal relationships and cancer: A theoretical analysis. *Journal of Social Issues*, *35*, 120–155.

Wortman, C., & Silver, R. (1987). Coping with irrevocable loss. In G. VandenBos & B. Bryant (Eds.), *Cataclysms, crises, and catastrophes: Psychology in action* (pp. 189–235). Washington, DC: American Psychological Association.

Zarling, C., Hirsch, B., & Landry, S. (1988). Maternal social networks and mother-infant interactions in full-term and very low birthweight, preterm infants. *Child Development*, *59*, 178–185.

Zitrin, A., Ferber, P., & Cohen, D. (1964). Pre- and perinatal factors in mental disorders of children. *Journal of Nervous and Mental Diseases*, *139*, 357–361.